MIRACLE BABY: AN ALTERNATIVE PREGNANCY

MIRACLE BABY: AN ALTERNATIVE PREGNANCY

Andrea L Duran-Carpenter

Carl Janicek

Dr. Stacey Maxfield

Deanna Romero

U.S. Copyright for book, "Miracle Baby: an Alternative Pregnancy"

Copyright © 2015 Andrea L Duran-Carpenter & Carl Janicek & Dr. Stacey Maxfield & Deanna Romero
All rights reserved.

ISBN: 1494297124
ISBN 13: 9781494297121

AUTHORS'/PUBLISHER'S NOTE

Please note this book is not a substitute for medical advice and understand that when implemented, you are engaging in this process at your discretion. This my personal story about how I achieved a successful pregnancy. The authors, and the publisher of this book are not responsible for anything that can or could go wrong; there are no warranties and no guarantees that the process will work for you and your situation. The authors of this book encourage all readers to consult with trained medical professionals, homeopaths/naturopaths, spa professionals, chiropractors and acupuncturists to aid in conception. Please hire trained certified professionals with the necessary board certifications and that they can provide recommendations from highly credible sources. Verify their background with your local Better Business Bureau and regulators of your state's licensed medical professionals. Always communicate only, with professionals about your treatments, goals, and expectations.

I dedicate this book to my family, my friends,
my miracle baby—my daughter, "Aly," and to God.

CONTENTS

    Authors'/Publisher's Note v
    Preface xi
    Acknowledgements xiii
1. The final third pregnancy: Birth at Last 3
2. Pregnancy 1: Molar Pregnancy 6
3. Pregnancy 2: Preparation and Miscarriage: 9
    Liver Cleanse 9
    Herbal Wrap 12
    Chiropractic/Acupuncture 14
    Miscarriage Two 17
    Neuro-energetics/Balanced Health 18
4. Homeopathic Process-Carl Janicek 23
5. Men's Health by Carl Janicek 43
6. "Third Time is a Charm:" Beginning of a Successful Pregnancy: 54
    First Trimester:
    Month 1: 54
    Month 2: 57
    Month 3: 58
7. Second trimester 59
    Month 4: 59
    Month 5: 59
    Month 6 60
8. Third Trimester 62
    Month 7 62
    Month 8 65
    Month 9 66
9. Conclusion 68

Appendix · 73
Index · 77
Bibliography · 79
About The Authors · 81

PREFACE

I waited many years to have children. As you will read, when I finally decided to become a mother, I did have a bit of a struggle. In this book, I will share how I achieved a successful pregnancy. I believe this process will be most effective for women in their 30's to early 40's.

First, after reading this book, written by Toni Weschler, M.P.H., *"Taking Charge of Your Fertility: the Definitive Guide to Natural Birth Control, Pregnancy Achievement, and Reproductive Health,"* I thought to myself, "I have nothing to lose and I will try this!" I found the segment in the book about alternative medicine for pregnancy to be particularly inspiring. Soon after reading this book, another colleague referred me to a chiropractor/acupuncturist. Then my friend, who is a physician's assistant, recommended the Liver cleanse for balancing the body and later, she referred me to a doctor of Homeopathy.

Second, the book, *"The Secret"* inspired me to write, *"Miracle Baby: an Alternative Pregnancy."* The authors said, "When we are positive in our thought process, our thoughts become our reality." Soon I began to see myself as being pregnant, and, in time, my pregnancy became a reality. The day after day, I would say the Saint Ann prayer, visualizing a healthy pregnancy, and how it would feel to touch and hold my baby in my arms. I kept saying to myself, "I will not be denied the beautiful experience of having my child, and no one will tell me that I am too old! I can do this!"

Third, I am a woman who believes in making intelligent, responsible, informed choices and the need to avoid invasive medical procedures. The method described in this book can cost about $6,000 a year. In most cases, this should be the total expense, but for some, more treatments, and more expense, may be required. A colleague once said to me, "It is sad that people have this knowledge and don't share this information with the public." So, while I could keep this information confidential and to myself, I have decided to share my experience with you so that you might also be successful in your vision.

In summary, it is my view that to withhold information that would potentially benefit other women is not a choice I would make. The cost of this method is minimal, particularly when compared to a daughter's love and laughter. I highly recommend reading, *"The Secret."* If we were to analyze successful people, we would find they have the power to overcome adversity, by living and visualizing success in their everyday lives.

ACKNOWLEDGEMENTS

There are many influential people, who knowingly and unknowingly helped create this book:

I want to thank a past colleague named Dawn. When we worked together as travel agents, we would discuss alternative supplements, aromatherapy, and acupuncture. She is the one who said to me, "Amazing, people know this, and don't share this with the public." So, Dawn--this book is for you!

I also want to thank Deanna Romero, a physician's assistant, a friend, a healer, a Curandera, (Spanish for medicine woman), an avatar, and co-author of this book. I am deeply grateful and appreciate all of her support. Deanna gave me the courage and knowledge to understand my body. She helped me see the bright side of my previous miscarriages, and to understand what it means to balance the body. She is one incredible "Curandera!"

I owe a lot to Dr. Stacey Maxfield. If it wasn't for her expertise, I might have had a total of six miscarriages and still not have my precious daughter, Aly. Dr. Maxfield helped me to remain focused, and she repeatedly informed me about how important acupuncture and chiropractic adjustments were to achieve pregnancy. Again and again, she will go the extra mile for her patients. In August of 2012, Dr. Maxfield died from cancer. Thank you, for everything, Dr. Maxfield!

Carl Janicek, a doctor of homeopathy, showed me the importance of cleansing my body, eating nutritional foods, and adding proven and appropriate fortifying supplements to my diet. He made me realize "three lattes a week" can be deadly to both your liver and your livelihood. He opened the gateway for my child's birth, and I thank him, for all of his help and support. Thanks, for everything!

I also want to credit my obstetrician and gynecologist, and her entire team of professionals, for believing, "The third time is a charm." Thank you, Dr. Monica Abarca, for being there for my journey!

Lastly, this book is dedicated to every woman out there who has the desire to become a mother and for all mothers. In this book, I will share how I achieved a successful pregnancy. It is my hope that after reading this book, each of you will know how to have a very healthy and successful pregnancy. Good luck and God, bless all of you future moms!

THE JOURNEY

THE FINAL THIRD PREGNANCY: BIRTH AT LAST

Finally, after two unsuccessful pregnancies! I called the hospital at 8:00 p.m. on November 6, 2006, but my room wasn't ready. It was planned induction into the pregnancy hall of fame. I called a half hour later, and they said, "Your room will be ready at about 9:30 p.m." I was so excited; it was time!

We arrived at the hospital, filled out all the paperwork, went to the maternity ward and gave the nurse my birthing plan accompanied by a box of chocolates, for her and her colleagues.

TIP: I highly recommend a birthing plan accompanied by a box of chocolates or a basket of fruit for the nurses, doctors, and all personnel. They will be working very hard for you, so treat them with a high regard when necessary. Please Google, Bing, or Zoo for a birthing plan.

So, as soon as we were settled, I received medication to end the journey. I awoke at about 8:00 a.m. the next day and my water was broken. I was given Oxytocin (Pitocin) to boost my contractions. A nurse came into my room about an hour later to check the dilation. I thought to myself, "Is this when I am supposed to forget my dignity, is this when I am supposed to lose my shyness?" I dilated to something like 3.5 cm, and I still can't push. Every time I was touched, I felt swollen inside. Another check showed a dilation of 7.5 cm. At about 1:00 p.m. in the dilation was 9.3 cm, can I push? I think not! Good Lord, I feel like a bloated puffer fish! It hurts! It hurts! Relax and breathe! Relax and breathe! I vocalize loudly, "Epidural please!" I wanted to do everything natural, but the pain was intense. Natural isn't for everyone! The experience reminded me of the song from the 70's (or the lyric) that was titled, "I am woman, do ya hear me roar," by the artist Helen Reddy. Instead I thought, "I am woman--do you hear me scream!" Oh, God!

She arrived around 3:00 p.m.--my miracle baby, "Aly," and the doctor said, "Happy birthday, baby!" I didn't see her right away because of the C-section, and I was still heavily sedated from the epidural. I looked to my right and thought that must be my doctor.

No. It was my husband with our baby girl, "Aly." At that moment, I thought back to the beginning of my journey and my eyes were filled with tears. So, maybe your journey started like mine, or maybe your situation is just a bit different than mine. I had had two miscarriages in my late 30's, and by this point I realized I needed more help to sustain a healthy pregnancy. I needed to balance my entire body and to balance my hormones.

I saw my friend, Deanna Romero for a treatment during my second miscarriage. I needed Neuroenergetics to relax my body. This method of acupuncture is great because it works to eliminate the need for C-sections. Unfortunately, I did need a C-Section and Deanna was not present at the delivery. But what made me consider the various methods of acupuncture is the fact it has existed for thousands and thousands of years in Asia.

Also, regarding my second miscarriage, I saw the chiropractor/acupuncture/nurse two months before the second miscarriage. The chiropractor said in my third pregnancy, to come in during my seventh-month adjustment and acupuncture to prevent birth defects.

During my third and successful pregnancy, I saw Carl and Dr. Maxfield. Carl suggested cleansing my body again, but specifically the intestines. The intestines absorb nutrients, so it was imperative to get them functioning properly. While working with Carl, I learned I needed to take natural supplements, to eat healthier foods, to rest and to exercise for a successful pregnancy. In other words, I had to ramp up my body for my "Miracle Baby!"

I changed my diet for pregnancy, for the rest of my life, and for my child's life. I used to eat junk food about 50 percent of the time, or food of no nutritional value. So, I started eating more raw fruits, vegetables and freshly prepared foods a whopping 80 to 90 percent of the time. I also try to avoid foods cooked in a microwave, certain loaded chemical, frozen foods I can't even pronounce. I try to stay away from foods made with bleached flour and white sugar, high fructose, hydrogenated fats, and corn syrup. I now have 6 oz. White chocolate lattes only four times a year. I drank non-alcoholic beverages during my pregnancy. I now try to drink the standard amount of filtered water every day. I don't smoke. Again, I'm not perfect with my diet, so someone might occasionally see me eating a donut, but I only eat a donut once a month or not at all. I do believe in moderation.

PREGNANCY 1: MOLAR PREGNANCY

We conceived in November 2003. A month prior to getting pregnant, I spoke with female colleagues, and they said to purchase this book. The book is entitled, *"Taking Charge of Your Fertility: the Definitive Guide to Natural Birth Control, Pregnancy Achievement, and Reproductive Health,"* by Toni Weschler, M.P.H.

> **TIP: I highly recommend this book, "Taking Charge of Your Fertility."**
> **I read the revised edition published 2002, but you can check with your bookstore, or on the internet, for a more current copy.**

This book by Toni Weschler, M.P.H. covers several topics, including: "Fertility Awareness: What You Should Know and Why You Probably Don't, Taking Control of Your Reproductive Health, There's More to Your Reproductive Anatomy Than Your Vagina, Finally Making sense of Your Menstrual Cycle, The Three Primary Fertility Signs, and How to Observe and Chart Your Fertility Signs." Also, have your hormone levels checked as well as the functionality of your thyroid. My husband had his sperm count checked, and he wasn't too thrilled about this invasive test. Check with your doctor to see if your partner should have his thyroid checked. Author Toni Weschler, M.P.H., also discusses how to check your period and how to look at your discharges for fertility signs. This book has an appendix about, "Troubleshooting Your Cycle: Expecting and unexpected." It contains a very detailed glossary--an example is the term "molar pregnancy."

"Taking Charge of your Fertility", gives the definition of a molar pregnancy: "A rare condition in which a normal pregnancy goes awry, becoming a benign tumor at about ten weeks." Why is it important to know about a molar pregnancy? A molar pregnancy could have killed me! After ten weeks of being pregnant, my sister-in-law said to me, "Go to the doctor!" I was over the age of 35. After all I had been on the pill for 18 years; I didn't think there would be any problems. I am healthy; my mother didn't hit menopause until she was 50. My grandmother had my father when she was 39 years old. My first cousin had two children when she was between the ages 37 to 41.

> **TIP: Listen to your body after conception. Take note, my molar pregnancy immediately felt like a weed in a garden rapidly growing out of control. I craved nothing but Reese's Pieces, pickles and Top Ramen noodles. On the other hand, during my <u>normal pregnancy, I could feel</u> the embryo attaching to my womb. Then, within the first month I craved a more balanced diet. A woman should contact her doctor, nurse practitioner, or midwife as soon as she finds out she is pregnant.**

The nurse turned me on my right side, then the left side and even had another nurse come in and check for a heartbeat, there was nothing. Nothing! I thought what was wrong with my baby? Why can't she hear the heart beat? The nurse said, "We need to get an ultrasound." She left and came back stating she had scheduled it for the following morning.

That morning, I called work and was excused until 11:00 a.m. I walked in for the ultrasound, and the technician was friendly but had no comment about my baby. I asked, "Can I see my baby?" She turned off the machine and then said the machine was inoperative. I walked back to the office, and the receptionist called me up to the desk, handed me the phone, saying, "Your doctor's on the phone." The doctor said, "I'm afraid your pregnancy isn't going as we expected." I immediately drove to her office. Then, I called work and spoke with human resources, and they approved the rest of the day off. I was told I needed to fill out the necessary FMLA paperwork.

The doctor said, "We need to remove the pregnancy." She said if I didn't have the "D and C," I might need chemotherapy. The definition of a "D and C" from, *"Taking Charge of Your Fertility"* is a surgical procedure used to scrape the surface of the endometrium with an instrument called a curette. Prior to curettage, the cervix is gradually opened with instruments called dilators. I was also told after the "D and C," that my hormones must normalize or that I would need chemotherapy.

Then my doctor said for a month after the "D and C," I would need to have blood drawn once a week. The doctors said this was to make certain there were no remaining pieces of the tumor and that my hormone levels were declining. After a month of blood draws, she then ordered a blood draw once a month for an entire year. Great! Then she recommended that I shouldn't try to get pregnant for an entire year. How old would I be then? I would be 38 years of age. Damn it; why was this happening to me? I asked God, repeatedly, "Why I couldn't have my baby?" I cried out to girlfriends and colleagues by venting profusely. Then I rationalized, why not me?

Every female colleague who read, *"Taking Charge of the Your Fertility,"* was having a successful pregnancy, except for me. One colleague started talking to my boss about how ecstatic she was about having twins. Then she excused herself, and she said how sorry she was about my miscarriage. My employer accommodated every woman during her pregnancy. One woman had been on the job for seven years, but when she became pregnant, suddenly she started being abrupt, moody with customers, yet no one fired this woman. One of my supervisors told me to let her know when I was pregnant so she could allow me to take breaks when necessary. They took care of their employees. But with my next employer and my next pregnancies, there was very little accommodation. Produce! During this time of employment, I sought professionals in acupuncture, chiropractic treatments, homeopathy and balanced health with Neuroenergetics.

TIP: Know the law where you live because, in some states, such as Colorado, an employer doesn't have to accommodate pregnancy. Colorado is a hire and fire at will state.

PREGNANCY 2: PREPARATION AND MISCARRIAGE:

In January 2005, I had a new job, and I had started the Liver Cleanse. During this time, I used Neuroenergetics for balanced health. A colleague referred me to a chiropractor/acupuncturist who could help me achieve a successful pregnancy. I proceeded to have an herbal wrap and a miscarriage.

> **TIPS:** My definition of a Neuroenergetics is where a licensed professional touches body acupuncture pressure points with the touch of the fingertips, and then the patient may be asked to inhale or exhale breathing.
>
> A licensed, or trained spa professional will dip their hand or delicate brush into a cold, euphoric, and thick herbal paste. The spa expert smears sticky stuff on all body extremities. The bikini area is untouched. The professional wraps the body with plastic or bandages. The professional then walks you over to a treadmill, for some exercise.

LIVER CLEANSE

At that time, I started the Liver Cleanse to detoxify my body internally. Deanna my friend, who is a physician's assistant, recommended I should do the Liver Cleanse before attempting my second pregnancy.

> **TIP:** The ingredients of Cleanses change over time, and for the purpose of bettering our health. Check with a reputable Homeopath or Naturopath for a recommended cleanse. I specifically did the Liver

Cleanse for weight loss and a successful pregnancy and created by D. Gary Young, author of the cleanse book, *"Re-JUVA-nate Your Health."*

Deanna Romero, P.A. on the role of a Physician Assistant in the Liver Cleanse process:

I have known Andrea for several year, and she would come to me with questions about any health problem or questions she was having. I knew she wanted to get married and have a family, which she finally did. She became married, and the couple decided to have a family; however, she soon ran into problems with her first pregnancy experience, a "molar pregnancy." Then, her second pregnancy ended in a miscarriage.

We had a long talk, and I told Andrea she would benefit from doing a "liver cleanse" to bring her body into balance. Cleansing the liver is one of the most important cleanses one can do for the body, but not just any liver cleanse. The liver cleanse I was referring to was the one outlined by Dr. Gary Young with Young Living essential oils. It is called "Rejuvenate Your Liver." The cleanse is nutritionally based cleanse which detoxifies, rebuilds nutrition, alkalizes, and cleanses the colon as well. Also, improves immune function and is directed at the liver. It is more of a complete cleanse that creates an environment for detoxification of the liver. There are many different cleanses out there but, this cleanse is a complete cleanse, as if you were doing a spring-cleaning of your body.

The liver handles filtering and processing all foods, nutrients, drugs, alcohol, and other materials. The liver then lets them enter and pass through the blood stream to further break them down and store them. Also produces bile that breaks down fat. In addition, the liver plays a role in producing immune cells to help fight infection. It also produces proteins for blood coagulation and removes toxins and bacteria from the blood. Unfortunately, our body cannot break down non-organic chemicals to which we are exposed; therefore, they get stored in the fatty tissue of the liver and other fatty organs. The liver by far is where most chemicals and metals are stored, which in turn compromises liver function. The liver also plays a role in hormonal balance, breaking down cholesterol, testosterone, and estrogen.

The liver plays a role in the quality of every function that goes on in the body. It is like the core and anchor of our bodies. In addition, there is an important physiology the liver plays in our bodies since the liver is also the organ that stores anger and emotional traumas. This physiology gets down to a cellular level in which DNA replicates cellular memory that holds emotional imprints on our experiences. For all these reasons, now you start to get the idea of why it so important to have a healthy functioning liver. When the liver is damaged due to over-consumption of alcohol, hepatitis, poor diet, or chemical exposures, there is a spillover of toxins into the blood stream that create degenerative diseases. Cleansing the liver is the key to health and longevity. The "Rejuvenate your Liver" cleanse requires some discipline since it requires a combination of nutritional and dietary changes. The "Master Cleanse" drink is used in this cleanse, as are Vita Life, Juva Spice, Juvapower, Ningxia Red, which helps provide nutrition to live. There are essential oils included in the Juva Cleanse blend then break down metals, chemicals and help flush the liver. In addition to nutrients and detoxifying ingredients, there are enzymes used to break down fat and toxin. Lastly, there is the colon supplement, Comfortone, which is a good combination to use during "Master Cleansing." To get more details on this cleanse you can find additional information in the "Rejuvenate Your Liver" by Gary Young, at youngliving.com.

Results of cleansing your liver are amazing depending how you cleanse. You can cleanse for five days up to three months. After cleansing, your allergies will be eliminated for a month, which was my experience with Eczema. Your energy level and motivation will increase, and your sleep will improve. Weight loss continues the longer you cleanse, hormonal balance improves, and protein metabolism also improves. Emotions will be released, and any anger will clear, thus giving you a state of peacefulness and overall sense of well-being.

After Deanna had explained all this information to me, I was ready to take control of my health and get my body ready to conceive once again. But this time, I was determined to carry my baby to term. In addition, to making the recommendation to rejuvenate my liver, Deanna also referred me to Carl Janicek, a homeopathic doctor. I believed Dr. Janicek could help me have a healthy pregnancy and get my hormones balanced. I also believed my long-term use of oral contraception played a role in some of the problems I was experiencing. I told Deanna that my obstetric/gynecologist stated not to be surprised if I miscarried three more times before being able to carry a pregnancy to term. After hearing this, I was determined to have a healthy pregnancy, and I did what she believed would make the difference to have my miracle baby.

TIP: The beginning first few days of any cleanse, you may feel exhausted, nauseated or even dehydrated. A cleanse can be brutal! You may also feel lethargic. If you're worried about job performance, consider vacation time. A cleanse can be a week, 14 days or even longer. Clarify duration of cleansing with a doctor, or licensed professional.

HERBAL WRAP

In June 2005, I decided to have an "Herbal Wrap" after my sister-in-law told me that there were stories about women successfully getting pregnant following an herbal wrap. Then a colleague mentioned you can have two herbal wraps a year. I was skeptical. I believe there is more to getting pregnant, and I will try!

I went to an alternative gym that had exercise equipment, massage therapy, herbal wraps, alternative healing oils, and aromatherapy. I walked to the counter and said, I am here for my wrap." I went to the back room, and they asked me to leave the undergarments on my body. There they proceeded to apply this olive colored paste. It smelled heavenly! Then Ace bandages were wrapped all over my body and bandages right around the critical area for the conception, just under the belly button, but over the pubic hair line. I was determined to do whatever it took to stimulate my body for pregnancy.

TIP: Before having an herbal wrap if you have sensitive skin, think you might have allergies to herbs, or if you are taking medications, please contact a physician immediately. Check with your physician to find out if you can have this type of exercise herbal wrap. Also, remember that herbal wraps should be done twice a year. You should verify that your spa is professionally licensed with the Better Business Bureau in your area or ask for credentials, and recommendations. Again, check with your doctor, a licensed homeopath,

licensed naturopath, a licensed chiropractor, nurse, etc. Also, be sure to drink plenty of water before the wrap.

Behold, the mummy's sister! I was told to put on a plastic athletic sweat suit and lie down on a massage therapy table. My feet were elevated about six inches using a device that moved my feet back and forth for about 15 minutes. I then put on these a pair of comfortable athletic flip flops and followed them over to the treadmill.

The mummy's sister was off to the races, for a half hour! I kept looking at the clock and thinking, "I'm burning up--Houston, can you hear me? I'm in my exercise space suit." I thought to myself, "Will I have excellent results from this wrap? Hold the tortilla, please!" The perspiration was pouring out of my suit. The timer finally went ding. I had lost about a ¼ of an inch on every body extremity. I reminisced back to my college days, when my nutrition instructor, Candace, at Metropolitan State University Denver said, "Anytime we lose more than two pounds a week, we're losing water and not fat. Adequate weight loss is two pounds a week."

TIP: Remember adequate weight loss is two pounds a week. Anything above two pounds is usually water loss. Consult with your doctor. Detoxify your body and contact a credible Homeopath or Naturopath.

My skin felt pearly smooth, and suddenly I had this urge, and I started singing a song by K.C. and the Sunshine Band *titled Get down tonight."* But, what good is, *"Get down tonight?"* I was not ovulating, so I edited that thought right out of my mind! Yes, I left the gym!

Now, there are different types of herbal wraps. There is the mermaid herbal wrap, the exercise wrap that I mentioned, and the standard herbal greenish clayish wrap with ace bandages or saran wrap. Great strides can be made from exercise wraps.

About a week after doing the herbal wrap, I contacted the chiropractor/acupuncturist. A colleague of mine referred me to Dr. Maxfield and stated she is an excellent chiropractor/acupuncturist. How, and why, could she help me?

CHIROPRACTIC/ACUPUNCTURE

I was hesitant about seeing a chiropractor and having acupuncture treatments. Dr. Maxfield explained the process. She said there would be adjustments once a week and acupuncture for an entire month. Afterwards, I'd need monthly acupuncture and chiropractic adjustments up and until conception. I was reluctant, but it worked.

Dr. Maxfield—a brief autobiography

I would like to start with just a few notes about myself before we get into the real guts of how chiropractic and acupuncture work to allow the body to heal itself. I was born and raised in Des Moines, Iowa. I was an avid swimmer and did very well despite the fact that I had not found chiropractic. My father took a severance package from John Deere, the summer before my senior year and we moved to Texas. Thank God! I will get back to that statement.

I finished high school and immediately entered community college trying to figure out what I wanted to be when I grew up. After completing all of the basic courses, I decided to take the pre-med route. However at that time, I could not sit, stand, sleep, drive a car, or focus on my schoolwork. Anyone who has ever suffered through a bout of sciatica can understand.

I went to several doctors and ended up with an orthopedic surgeon. After X-rays and an MRI, he determined that I had a herniated disc. From there, his only suggestion was to perform a steroid epidural, which would hopefully bring relief. I ended up having that procedure done a total of three times. I understood that was the maximum amount of times such a procedure was allowed. The first two epidurals were like heaven. I received approximately three to four months of relief from each. The bad news did not arrive until I had the procedure a third time and got no relief at all. As a matter fact, I felt like I got hit by a truck. I was worse if you can believe that. Upon returning to the doctor, I received even more bad news. He did not feel that I was a surgical candidate. The reason he stated was that Swiss studies have proved back surgery usually only lends relief for approximately five to ten years and at the age of twenty-one, I was simply too young. While I hated that doctor on that day, I now praise God for him. He simply dismissed me and told me to find another outlet to get rid of the pain. Physical therapy was his only suggestion.

Left to my own devices, I decided to go the "quack" doctor, with the actual title: Doctor of Chiropractic. To my disbelief, after approximately eight visits, my pain was non-existent. The astonishing part was that he was not surprised at all. That coupled with the fact the seemed to love his career so deeply. It led me to want to finish my schooling in the realm of the healing arts, for no drug ever came close to making me feel as good as the chiropractor did.

You must still be wondering, why I was so happy to have relocated to Texas. As many of you know, Iowa has some of the best schools in the country--not to discount the quality of Texas schools. Those great schools come at a very high premium from a monetary standpoint. I cannot say at this point whether or not I, with the help of my parents, would have been able to afford higher education in Iowa. Although Texas had fabulous in-state tuition rates at all their state schools. So, I decided to continue with the pre-med route and eventually went on to get my doctorate from Parker College of Chiropractic in Dallas.

Due to the extreme heat and lack of outdoor activities, I chose to move to Colorado after I graduated and opened my practice. After I began practicing and saw the wonderful miracles of the human body could heal without interference, I decided to spend my continuing education hours furthering my knowledge of acupuncture. Eventually, I added that practice to my license. That was one of the best decisions; I could have ever made.

I have had many successes throughout my years in practice with both chiropractic and acupuncture. Due to privacy issues I can discuss some examples but must withhold any detailed information. In these writings, I will only deal with the cases of fertility. One of my first cases concerning fertility was before I had a license to practice acupuncture. I had been in practice for only a short time when I met a woman who was getting ready to have an in-vitro procedure. She had already tried the procedure once and had exhausted all of her extra finances. You will hear this again, but she explained due to her financial strain that this was her last shot. Just having the knowledge of anatomy and what happens to that anatomy when interference is removed, I felt I could help her in this process. The third lumbar vertebrae in the spine innervate the sex organs, so that is where I concentrated the majority of my efforts during her treatments. Considering the fact a pinched spinal nerve will not allow proper function of the sex organs proved to be true. After removing all interference regarding that nerve, her procedure was successful. She now has very lovely children.

The next case that came to me was a young lady who had also tried in-vitro unsuccessfully.

This time it was much scarier for me because she had the procedure done four times with no success. Once again, I was told this was her last try not only due to the financial burden but due to the emotional stress the lack of success was having on both her and her husband. By this time, I had learned the acupuncture prescription that aids with fertility issues. This meant I had two weapons to fight whatever was preventing the in-vitro process from working. Once again, all was successful, and she also has two lovely young children.

My third case is the one that makes me a true believer of the balance that can be achieved within the human body. Another young lady came to me, (I was now getting many referrals with fertility issues), before an in-vitro process. She was distraught as you can guess as she had tried this once before and could only afford to this one last time. Over time, though, there were signs things were not going well. To this day, I can still remember the day she came to my office in tears and told me the doctor had informed her things did not look very well. For any of you who have had or tried to have children, you can understand how devastating this news must have been to her. They were not sure any of the embryos would be viable but were going to go ahead with the transfer. All I could do was reassure her that her body was in balance now and ready this to conceive. Everything was successful, and she now has three lovely children. Now, before you get too concerned and think this is tabloid material, she had one child with the procedure I just discussed. Then she had her twins with another procedure that I helped her with a couple of years later.

Lastly, I will discuss Andrea's case. She came to me as a "forty-something" who had a molar pregnancy and wished to become pregnant again. Everything I could remember from my embryology class many years back told me a pregnancy of this type was very rare. One thing I was certain of is that a molar pregnancy always resulted in miscarriage due to lack of substance. Andrea was also very adamant about using holistic measures to achieve her dream of becoming a mother.

With the use of chiropractic and acupuncture, as well as other holistic work, she easily became pregnant. But to both of our disappointment, she had a miscarriage.

I do remember at the time Andrea was under a great deal of stress from her job. At this point, all things had to be considered. Many things could have caused this mishap, but one must consider the health of the body from different angles. Were there hormonal imbalances due to age, or even her long-term use of birth control pills? I wondered what type of nutrition was being fed to her body and was supplementation necessary? I was also concerned about her state of mind during that period considering all of the stress she was under. After considering all of this, we proceeded again with acupuncture and spinal manipulation. She came in for treatment twice a week at first and then once a week until conception. This time was different, though. We had both learned a valuable lesson. She learned she must take care of her body and her mind. I learned that I must treat a patient vigorously all the way through her first trimester. I also learned there must be a wellness check further into a pregnancy to keep everything moving along smoothly. Bringing the mind and body into balance was the key to success in Andrea's case. While she did all of the work to remove interference within her body, outside forces can also be praised for allowing this miracle to happen.

MISCARRIAGE TWO

Was it a success at last? No--it was another miscarriage. My heart was pounding rapidly! I changed jobs and took on even more stress. I was unaware at the time how stressful this position would be, with attrition everywhere. It followed this employer's high expectations for good performance with little pay, minimal training, and no managerial support. It was career suicide! My boss kept saying, "You're an excellent employee, now go do more!"

I didn't realize I was pregnant. Certain smells made me nauseous, such as burnt popcorn that I could smell 25 feet away. Every situation became amplified as though someone had turned up the volume. Then the realization came--Mother Nature didn't greet me with her monthly visit. I informed human resources about my pregnancy, and there was no assistance. I wanted to make certain I had a normal pregnancy, so I contacted my physician, and a blood draw was scheduled to check hormone levels. I was exhausted and argumentative. There was no escaping these hormonal changes.

I continually found myself acting irrationally all day long, even yelling at my boss. I was out of control. I kept saying to myself, "Thank you, God, for ending this day!" Suddenly, I didn't feel like my normal self. Something was wrong. I felt decompression, like a balloon letting out air. Stress was doing this! I was in denial. Can stress cause birth defects? Can stress cause miscarriage?

TIP: Beware of what stress can do to your body and unborn child. A good source of information before conception and when dealing with high levels of stress is the book titled, "The Fertility Diet," by Jorge E. Chavarro, M.D., ScD and Walter C. Willett, M.D., Dr. P.H.

The following evening I received a call from the doctor who told me, "Your hormone levels aren't where we'd like them to be." She then asked me to schedule an ultrasound. The call disconnected, and I kept repeating in my mind, "What does she mean my pregnancy isn't going the way she'd like?"

I had an ultrasound the seventh week of pregnancy. I saw this blob, a circle, and there was a heartbeat of 110 heart beats per minute. I was expecting to see a head and a body, not a circular blob. This was a sign of heartache! I'm a failure!

TIP: I learned that a healthy heartbeat should be between 160 beats per minute to 180 beats per minute. Check this out with your physician, nurse practitioner, or midwife.

The ultrasound ended, and a technician said, "Please have a seat in the waiting area." The nurse called my name. The doctor was positive about hearing the heartbeat and informed me that we weren't out of the woods.

NEURO-ENERGETICS/BALANCED HEALTH

I went home, but because I wasn't doing the Kegel exercise correctly, I managed to get a bladder infection. The doctor's office called back on my urine sample. I also had a yeast infection, and I proceeded to take over the counter medication. At this time, I contacted my friend Deanna Romero, a physician assistant, to explain my frustration. I made an appointment to see her. I went to her office and paid for a Neuroenergetics (N.E.R.) treatment.

Statements by Deanna Romero, Physician Assistant:

Some work I performed with Andrea that may have had an impact on getting her balanced physically and hormonally was Neuroenergetic Release. The vast majority of people have a core distortion in their posture, which is held in place energetically via the tonus regulating system. Health is balance and is balance health. I had given Andrea a series of treatments before she conceived, and it is my belief there are a higher number of C-sections in this country based on the anatomical misalignment of the pelvis.

I recently was able to put this to test with one of my cousins who had a pretty significant anterior tilt to her pelvis. I told her when it was time to deliver her baby; I wanted to be there so we could some work to get her hips balanced. I just spontaneously arrived at her house one evening when her daughter said, "My mom is upstairs; she is not feeling well." I went up there, and she told me she had been having Hick's contractions for several hours, but they were coming more frequently and lasting for a minute or so. After being there about an hour, I noticed they were coming every three to five minutes lasting about a minute. I said to her, "Are you sure these are not real contractions." She was not too sure, and she was not interested in going to the hospital and then getting sent home with false labor. She had been to the doctor two days prior and had him strip her membranes. She dilated to two cm. And 70 percent effaced at that time. He said, "Could you go to sleep with this?" She responded, "No." He said, "Go check yourself into the hospital to be evaluated."

As she arrived and was given a room, the nurse came in to examine her, and she was still at two cm. dilated and 70% effaced. As soon as the nurse left I said, "Ok, let's get to work." So I did some distance N.E.R. with her, and as I completed working on her lower back and hips, the contractions immediately came on with a vengeance. As we watched the intensity of the contractions on the monitor, her face told the story that things had progressed to another level. The nurse returned to the room and said, "Ok." She then directed my cousin to go for a walk after which she would recheck her. The nurse said, "If she does not progress, we will have to send her home." My cousin said, "I don't know, if I could walk with these contractions, they're strong." I said, "Well, let's give it a try."

She maybe lasted about ten minutes and was too uncomfortable. I told the nurse that she better check her. Well, she had dilated to five cm. and was 100% effaced. Now, it was a big rush to get her up to a delivery room. Her contractions were steady and hard, so I just worked with her by having her breathe and concentrate on letting the baby move down through her pelvis. She wanted an epidural and was waiting for the anesthesiologist. It took about another thirty minutes for the anesthesiologist to arrive and get prepped. By this time, she had progressed to ten centimeters. What surprised me was she did not weep, scream, nor lose her composure, not one time during this short, rapid progression of labor. It was quite amazing to see the end product of a beautiful life being born into our world without much trauma.

I believe that technology, which is able to monitor fetal heart tones that go up or down when babies are distressed, leads to more C-sections. It is very stressful on babies to push their way through a tilted and twisted pelvis that can lead to a longer delivery, which creates more stress on the baby and mother. Personally, since I have had two C-sections, which I believe were due to issues, I had with scoliosis. Now, that my core distortion pattern has been brought into balance with N.E.R., I know I would be able to deliver a baby vaginally. Although, usually a woman is not allowed to have a vaginal birth if she has had a history of having more than one C-section.

The man who developed the N.E.R. is also, working on collecting data on how N.E.R. makes a difference in fertility with women. Health is balance and balance is health. The musculoskeletal system directly affects the visceral organs in the body. I am grateful that Andrea allowed me to assist in the creation of the new life; she has brought into this world. Andrea was proactive in her goal, to become a mother and I believe that there was a way to defeat the odds, and she did.

TIP: Check with your doctor regarding the Kegel exercise.

I was stressed out and depressed about the results. Deanna proceeded to do N.E.R. or Neuroenergetics, which is a procedure that involves touching acupuncture without needles, just touching with thumbs and index fingers on the various pressure points. In my opinion, Neuroenergetics would be great for any woman in labor/delivery whose hips aren't aligned naturally. This procedure could reduce the need for C-sections and lawsuits.

This methodology uses meridians. As we progress through my journey, notice treatments of acupuncture and homeopathy utilizing meridians. The treatments I received from Deanna, Carl, and Dr. Maxfield all contributed to my successful pregnancy.

Now, Deanna discussed past treatments and suggested it was great that I did the Liver Cleanse back in January 2005. Instead of doing it for seven days, she said I should try it for 14 days. My next cleanse lasted ten days. Deanna stressed the importance of cleansing to detoxify your organs, prepare for the pregnancy, and heal one of the most important organs of all--the liver. She also advised me to start using Ninja Red product and to consider the usage of the hormonal supplements: Prenelone and Progessence made by Young Living and by D. Gary Young, N.D.

The following day, I saw the dreaded spot of blood. I told my husband, and he immediately rushed me to the hospital. The doctor called in the ultrasound technician, and he proceeded to do a pelvic exam. How I wished, he was my Obstetrician! Ugh! I wanted to run away! I wanted to go home! I don't want to be here, and I didn't want to hear bad news!

In comes the ultrasound technician with a wheelchair asking me if I'd like a warmed blanket. I said, "Sure." She did the ultrasound, and the heartbeat had dropped to 80 beats per minute. I thought, "When will it happen, when will we have our child?"

My husband and I waited and waited. The doctor said the mild bleeding was possibly caused by the placenta adjusting to the pregnancy. He said to contact my Obstetrician first thing in the morning, which I did.

I arrived at work and immediately contacted my personal Obstetrician's office. I spoke with the nurses, and they said to come in right away. I then asked my boss to be excused for my doctor's appointment, again with minimal accommodation.

The same nurse who discovered my molar pregnancy caught this miscarriage. She again brought out their low powered ultrasound machine. There was no heartbeat! She told me to come in tomorrow for the high-powered ultrasound. I thought to myself, "How many ultrasounds do I need? Am I through yet? Not!"

So, I had my fourth ultrasound. There was just a circle there with no heartbeat. I saw my Obstetrician, and she told me I was scheduled for a "Dilatation and Curettage," (D & C), on Monday afternoon.

So when Monday came, there I was at the hospital, again. The nurse handed me my stylish "Victoria Secret's"--you know, those sexy gauzy, stylish hospital briefs—not! I saw my doctor, the same one who did the prior "D & C" for my first miscarriage, and I told her, "The third time is a charm!" I told all of the doctors and nurses, "I will be back!"

A couple days later I called Deanna to ask her to recommend a Homeopath. She said to contact Carl Janicek. Deanna and I both knew I needed a little bit more help to sustain a viable pregnancy. I needed to balance my entire body and get mentally prepared.

HOMEOPATHIC PROCESS–CARL JANICEK

During the drive to Carl's mountain office, I noticed the view was breath taking. I walked into Carl's office; he shook my hand, and I sat down. He proceeded to explain the meridians of our body. Then he showed me this device that allowed him to determine, by simply touching specific points on my hand and foot if my body was balanced. He explained how to interpret the readings on the machine's gauge. For example, my intestines were below 45, which meant my intestines weren't functioning properly. If the intestinal score was over 55, that was normal. I had readings taken from my hand and foot, the meridians, and acupuncture pressure points. He also suggested I should use supplements, change my diet, and gave the reasons for these changes.

Carl Janicek's testimony:

My homeopathic experience started back in the 70's. With my father's encouragement, I used to see Hanna Kroeger, in Boulder, and Hanna ended up working with me. However, I didn't have much of an opinion about it, and I hesitated to pursue study in her school because I simply wasn't very open-minded. I had heard a lot of good things about Hanna, and her work, so my curiosity was at least tuned into what I might be able to learn. I heard so many things that sounded impossible, yet I continued to be at least interested in holistic methods. Both of my grandmothers used herbs to bring me back to health when I was a youngster, so I knew there was something of value in that path. I also believed natural healing was more spiritually aligned with healing on a deeper level that synthetic industrial methods could not touch. I experimented here and there, working with tissues, salts, and flower remedies.

I also had the opportunity to work at Craig Hospital in Englewood, Colorado. There, I had the chance to learn a great deal about current medical models being used in rehabilitation work, patient care, physical therapy, occupational therapy, speech therapy, and emergency procedures. I became interested in pursuing the study of physical therapy Plus, I liked doing hands-on patient care, which started me on the path of going to massage therapy school. There I found a few fantastic teachers who inspired me to an even greater appreciation of the mind-body-spirit combination.

NATURAL HEALTH AND HEALING

Unfortunately, there was little appreciation for that holistic model of healing at the hospital, where I was working. After having a motorcycle accident, I felt insulted by the emergency room care that I was given. At that point I realized I would have to find my way into this area of health and wellness that seemed, so obvious yet had an elusive quality that called to me and my spirit.

In the 70's, I had worked briefly with homeopathy just to see if it had any value. I also studied Martial arts under Sifu Ron Rosen, who was knowledgeable about Chinese Medicine, and who went on to become a well-known Traditional Chinese Medicine professor at several different schools. During this period many people thought Chinese medicine was hogwash. However, I became very convinced of the power and wisdom of understanding energy systems of the body, through my personal experiences, including the intimate relationship. We humans have with nature, all of our surroundings, as well as our personal choices.

I then went on to study acupuncture in more I depth with Dr. Eric Tao O, Md. After 1200 hours of classes, I decided putting needles into people was not my first choice of how I would spend my time. I didn't realize whatever I did, it would include those philosophies and tools of Chinese medicine. I was enthralled about learning more and more about this field. I had completed many classes, studied with many great practitioners, gained knowledge and training, but I felt like my studies were not complete. So, I pursued and received a Bachelor of Science degree in Wellness Nutrition, a pastoral degree. I did not feel like I wanted to start a church or become devoted to promoting a specific religious group. During this period, I met Dr. William Nelson N.D., an influential genius, who encouraged me to take a deeper view--a scientific view of homeopathy.

I wasn't sure I would like it. I was quite skeptical. But, as he patiently answered so many of my questions, and I had the opportunity to experience homeopathy first hand, I became completely entranced by the power of this misunderstood modality. I continued and studied his teachings, finally receiving a Doctorate in Homeo-therapeutics. For me, this was a new beginning, and I wasn't out of school for very long before I became aware of yet another powerful modality of natural healing. The power of Aromatherapy and Essential oils made from plants by a little company dedicated to purity and effectiveness. It was called, "Young Living Essential Oils," and founded by another man who seems way ahead of his time, Gary Young. Little did I understand at that time what a profound difference this knowledge and experience would make in my life, and on the lives of so many other people?

CARL'S DISCUSSION OF ANDREA'S VISITS

Her Visit--August 2005:

Andrea arrived at my office, and we talked about meridians and the device that was used, Tsing point technology, also known as Electro-Dermal Reactivity Screening (EDS). This device helps develop a deeper understanding of the energy systems of the body, similar to biofeedback from EEG or EKG.

I checked the meridians for balance in her entire body. I also spent time learning the words and images she held in her mind. I observed her mannerisms, limiting beliefs, and expressions. I asked about her blood type, her likes, and dislikes, and the nature of any complaints she had, as well as what times, made her feel better or worse. I took in as much information about her as possible in the intake appointment. Totality is the term in homeopathy. Much more time is spent listening to a client and to decide upon the actual core of the case. I asked her, "What is your goal with homeopathy," and she responded, "To sustain a viable pregnancy." Then we looked at symptoms she might be experiencing regarding her emotional, mental, and physical states. The data collection is a compilation known as "Totality of symptoms and synthesis."

Tsing point technology tests the "deep well" of the meridians by using Galvanic Skin Response and resistance giving an indicator of inflammation or degeneration.

Other methods of information collection can also be done by taking pulses and observing the tongue along with other clues.

Meridians relate to the function of the lymph nodes, large and small intestines, nervous system, circulatory system, triple warmer, gonadic organs, (testes, ovaries), adrenals, pituitary, thyroid, heart, pancreas, spleen, liver, cartilage, joints, stomach, fibrotic tissue, skin, essential fatty acid assimilation, gall bladder, and kidneys. Regarding the relations of meridians, Homeopathy, and Chinese medicine are in agreement on the doctrine of vitality and that the biggest difference between a healthy living body and a dead body isn't just its chemistry. **The biggest difference between a live and dead body is its energy, not its chemistry.**

DESCRIPTION OF A HOMEOPATHIC INTAKE AND TSING POINTS

During my Intake sessions, I conduct a homeopathic and nutritional evaluation along with a comprehensive interview process. This process includes taking readings from Tsing Points which are gathered and charted. If they are 40, it indicates a de-vitalization, or degeneration is at hand. If an "indicator drop" is observed then an active degenerative process could be attacking a person's system relating to the meridians. These meridian imbalances can be caused by some factors, most often toxicity from internal or external sources, or pathogenic infections, even at a low level. The degenerative readings can also be caused by radiation, microwaves, excess heat or cold, the wind, the noise, geopathic influences, or negative emotional states. The Chinese often call these sometimes subtle unseen disturbances, perverse energy. These energies can cause diseases, various cancers, systemic immune deregulation, Multiple Sclerosis, or other systemic deregulations, hypertension, or thyroid problems.

If the reading is within five points of 50 or around 50, this indicates a good balance of the meridian flow, noting that energy must be in a flow to be healthy. Any dam or blockage to an energy flow creates an imbalance both upstream and downstream and affects the meridian energy flows accordingly. Please see attached **Appendix** for better defining the **Flow and Pathways of Disease.**

The accuracies of this type of testing depend on a multitude of factors, including to a large extent, the experience of the practitioner, and the type of device used. In my system, a 60 or higher would indicate an inflammatory process in the body. The Chinese call this an excess, or burning up of chi, the element of fire, and usually includes the utilization of extra essential fatty acids, as well as other critical nutrients. The burning of chi is nearly always associated with an active inflammatory pathology. This excess reading can be very predictive of the disease process in an early phase, ultimately relating to a degenerative process that can be severe and have dire consequences, including death. This inflammation creates the fire and then ashes. An example of an inflammatory process would be arthritis (swollen joints, which usually ends its course with degeneration of the involved tissues. It is useful to note most diseases include an unregulated state of inflammation, mucous, and acidic bodily fluids that result in cellular stress, malnutrition, oxygen starvation, mutation, and even death.

Indicators of balance readings are in the range of 45 to 55. A few dietary items that can cause inflammation and set the stage for degeneration are excessive amounts of coffee, soda pop, and modified sugars like high fructose and corn syrup. However, in blood type "O," the genetic signatures from certain food sources such as wheat and corn, can be highly reactive to a person's immune response and can cause not only inflammation, but also can be a major factor in weight gain. I have found that every blood type is unique in its dietary reactivity, thus the book, "Eat Right for 4 Your Type," is useful and accurate most of the time. Therefore, it is well worth studying for anyone who wants to know more about his or herself, and about proper diet. Of course, our uniqueness as individuals and our specific traits play into who we are physically, emotionally, and constitutionally. Our uniqueness also goes far beyond the blood types that contribute to our immune responses and allergic reactions. Blood types are only one way to learn something about oneself.

LIFESTYLE HABITS AND CHOICES

I then had a discussion with Andrea to understand her lifestyle habits. We talked about how many items, such as some foods, dental work, exposure to food additives, chlorine, fluorine, fluoride, (which is being used less and less today since toxicity data continues to show damage to thyroid and other organ systems), industrial pollutants, smoke from tobacco, drugs, (both over the counter and prescribed), paints, plastics, insecticides and herbicides, metallics, petroleum and plastic residues, (such as those found in many bottled waters), pollutants in coffee machines, out-gassing from copy machines and paper products and other electronic devices, as well as carpeting, can all cause significant damage to the body including the unborn human fetus.

Some older computers using high emitting video displays also pose a risk from electrical radiation and iconic positive charges. Our culture and our economy thrive on products like these, as well as industrial petrol products, like gasoline and other carbon-based fossil fuels. Also, consider the Xenobiotic influences (toxic) which are available outside us that we may think are good for us due to advertising and promotional efforts by big pharmaceutical and agricultural corporations. Advertising often pushes these synthetic chemicals: acetaminophen, non-steroid inflammatories, insecticides, and herbicides-- all of which attack the reproductive system. In many situations, we are better off using carbohydrates rather than hydrocarbons.

I also screened Andrea for large parasites, or as I call it, the 800-pound gorilla in the corner of the room. Some folks don't like to talk about this. Anemotod, or worms that can damage the heart, brain, liver and other organs, are more common than most people realize. They can have a low-level negative effect on the host for many years. Often, too much time passes until the problem is discovered to be truly dangerous. Then it is only diagnosed after a period of stress or trauma to the system. Most often, people think of parasites having an effect on digestive organs, but they can attack many different organs and travel to nearly any part of the body.

Parasites have a life cycle that varies according to their family type and often have a relationship to the cycles of the moon. Modern industrialized medical methods may treat this hidden Gorilla type infestation. After treatment, the body may still be out of balance, and all too often treatment is incomplete. What I suggest, in this case, after the proper homeopathic nosode is given, is a course of pro-biotic therapy, and a much-needed intervention. I suggest Young Living "Life 5," which is a combination of five beneficial bacteria for the digestive tract. "Life 5" is a balanced and synergistic living gut flora, implanted in the intestines by daily use prior to going to bed. It is the active ingredient in the product that allows creation and absorption of proper nutrients.

TIP: "Life 5", may no longer be available. Please consult a professional for upgraded product.

When there is an imbalance of flora, (this can also happen due to lack of high-quality water), too much or not enough bile can be produced by the liver and an allergic reaction to particular foods can occur. Also, any irritation to the digestive tract can leave an area inflamed, allowing blood to come in contact with food, which stimulates an immune response, often thought of as a "food allergy." Most gallbladder pain and inflammation issues are a result of food reactivity.

In people with blood type "O's," as stated in the book, "Eat Right for 4 Your Type," by Dr. Peter J. Adamo, wheat and corn can cause constipation. This blood type turns corn and wheat carbohydrates, and other nutrients from these and many grains into adipose tissue (fatty tissue), to store toxins and may produce a compartmentalized type of fatty tissue in the body, better known as cellulite. A change of diet and proper massage techniques utilizing products like Young Living's Cellulite Magic can reduce cellulite dramatically.

HOMEOPATHIC REMEDIES

When bringing the body into balance, it is possible to use homeopathic drainage remedies to spill out, push, or drain the toxins. Homeopaths usually consider these to be shallower remedies. They treat a limited aspect of the person, in some ways similar to modern medical activities, and do not treat the constitution of the person as a whole. Whatever the philosophical and practical differences are, these drainage remedies are useful to bring the person into better health, out of suffering and even save his or her life. Drainage remedies made of herbs, xenobiotics, (toxic substances) and mid-range potencies of homeopathic remedies can be used as expellers. However, a great deal of expertise is required to choose the proper SAFE remedy and potency. In my personal experience, there is no substitute for the proper constitutional remedy when properly used.

Since homeopathy is constantly under attack by the pharmaceutical industry that spends millions of dollars in misinformation, it is best to understand better homeopathic practice and pharmacology. In creating a homeopathic remedy, the laboratory goes through a process of dilution and succession, which strengthens the original "Mother mixture" or actual source of the remedy such as a flower, herb, mineral, venom or even an insect. This process of dilution makes the original tincture less molecular in nature, and the process of successions makes medicine more energetically potent, while taking out the otherwise toxic nature of some materials. The process reduces its molecular weight and concentration in each progressive dilution, usually, in water and alcohol. The parts of alcohol, water, and remedy, can be varied according to how many stages of dilution and succession have been used. A 1X potency would be nearly a mother tincture, with the dilution being 1 part of the source solution, diluted to 9 parts water and ethyl alcohol. A 2X or 12X would be a progressive serial dilution, 2 (2X) times or 12 (12X) times, with each dilution being less molecular and more energetic. Higher energetic states of a properly given remedy tend to make the remedy more active, often affecting the mind as well as the physical body.

Homeopathy is a "proven" medicine. In "proving" remedies, the unknown remedies are taken by homeopathic practitioners, with a specific process to prove the actions of a specific remedy. Substances and specific potencies are recorded, unknown to anyone but the proving leader and the homeopathic pharmacy. Each "prover" is supervised by an advocate observer. And as the homeopath becomes sick or disturbed, the un-needed remedy is taken away and as he returns to health, the details of the experiences are observed. Supervisors contact the prover and then record the data and observations sometimes several times a day, for six to eight weeks. Then they meet, in what is called "an extraction" or "experience meeting," to tabulate data and form rubrics. The remedy is not disclosed to a proving participant or their supervisor until after all the data is collected and compiled.

HISTORY OF HOMEOPATHY

The father of classical homeopathy was Samuel H. Lenham, who lived from 1753-1845. His classical treatise titled, "Organon of Medicine," is even today a master's course in homeopathic medical practice, and here are some of his views:

He discusses the mission of a physician in paragraph two, defining the idea of the cure, "The highest ideal of a cure is rapid, gentle, and permanent restoration of health, or removal and annihilation of the disease in its whole extent, in the shortest, most reliable, and most harmless way, with easily comprehensible principles.

In the "Organon of Medicine" paragraph nine states: "In the healthy condition of man, the spiritual vital force (autocracy), the dynamics that animate the material body (organism), rules with unbounded sway, and retains all the parts of the organism in one admirable, harmonious vital operation, as regards both sensations and functions, so that our indwelling reason-gifted mind can freely employ this living healthy instrument for the higher purpose of our existence."

The Organon goes on to say in paragraph 16: "Our vital force, as a spirit like dynamic, cannot be attacked and affected by injurious influences on the healthy organism caused by the external inimical forces that disturb the harmonious play of life, otherwise, than in a spirit like (dynamic) way, and in like manner, all such morbid derangements (diseases) cannot be removed from it by the physician in other way than by the spirit-like (dynamic) alternative powers of the serviceable medicines acting upon our spirit like vital force.." Homeopathy is a type of energy exchanged exchanged in nature, and a remedy can be seen as information, vibration, or imprint from its source. The best and properly given remedy is based on the totality of symptoms in the patient. And can be perceived by an unbiased observer, as well as based one in "proven" actions of a given appropriate remedy.

HERRING'S LAW OF CURE

A concept of homeopathy, "Herrings Law of Cure," was created by German homeopath Constantine Herring in 1830's and he launched homeopathy in America with four fundamental qualities of healing:

1. *Healing processes from the inside out, then from the deepest part of an organism to the outer part of an organism. That includes mental and emotional, as well as vital organs. An example would be extremities, such as skin, where the symptoms appear and the healing process ends.*

2. *Symptoms tend to appear and disappear in the reoccurring order of appearance. Healing tends to progress from upper to lower parts of the body.*

3. *This top-down concept of healing or the need for healing may rid the body of the rest of the symptoms. Toxins or symptoms that live will release first before the skin.*

4. *Most illnesses of recent experience leave the body first. Acute cold or flu from several weeks ago would leave before chronic asthma from 20 years ago.*

NUTRITION, THE GRANDFATHER OF HEALTH AND WEALTH

NingXia Red is a food based supplement is recommended along with additional remedies. It is a powerful antioxidant manufactured by Young Living Essential Oils. It aids in balancing PH levels in the body. Overly acidic conditions form mucus in and around cells creating inflammation, which is the first step towards degeneration. One of the essential food ingredients is the NingXia Wolfberry. Most berries are sweet treats and valuable for their antioxidant values. Some berries have broad health benefits, like blueberries and raspberries. NingXia Red from Young Living is a concentrated juice blend that has been helping thousands of people, find new health and vitality. A person would have to consume about $30 in organic produce to equal overall nutrient values found in two ounces of NingXia Red Juice. NingXia Red contains powerful fortifying nutrients, such as vitamin C, calcium, magnesium, potassium, and numerous glucosaccarides, as well as zeaxanthins, which are missing in the common modern diet and absolutely critical for healthy eyes. This nutrient dense juice along with the Young Living product known as, "Multi Greens," provides most of the basic nutrients needed for a healthy day, even to the point of warding off the common cold, as well as many other ailments.

In my family, the NingXia juice helps keep us healthy. During the winter months when the cold and flu tend to be going around, it also helps balance out blood sugar and increase stamina during our summertime and weekend warrior adventures. I have not found anything else so nutritionally easy, pleasant tasting or nutrient packed. And, in testing it on so many of my clients, it proves to be helpful a majority of the time! NingXia Red is a rare find!

PH BALANCE

The Ph balance in the body has to do with the level of acid or alkalinity in the body fluids, tissues, blood, and organs. In all cases, there is the ideal balance to Ph, or optimum health and longevity balancing acid conditions in the body. However, in some cases, over alkalinity is the problem. Tests of saliva and urine are not comprehensive or accurate enough to make for scientific food evaluations. These imbalances in "terrain" tend to lead to most degenerative forms of a disease. The condition can appear as stubborn forms of arthritis, lowered immunity, and a general breakdown of systemic health. Ph imbalances also contribute to a vast array of mental health issues and learning disabilities.

Most people are unaware of the critical balance a body must maintain in regards to pH. Ideal venous blood pH is 7.46. It is critical for the body to maintain this pH balance. PH balance can be affected by diet and exercise patterns, as well as by toxins and pathogens. The blood pH is so significant for overall health and the ability to regenerate tissues that the body will steal minerals from the bone structure, to gather enough minerals to balance the blood pH. Often the body can't keep up with the various imbalances and demands, so some tissues and organs become morbid. In addition, it's also worth stating, many symptoms common today such as: fatigue, unknown aches and pains, obesity, food cravings, lower immunity, hyperactivity, attention deficit disorder, indigestion, colitis, diarrhea/

constipation, urinary tract infection, fungal infection, some forms of cancer, premenstrual syndrome, bacterial infections, viral infections, yeast infections, cirrhosis of the liver, and fertility issues-- can all be attributed to unbalanced blood pH levels. Finding our ideal bio-balance can be tricky and requires professional study and dietary intervention.

Our body is much like a garden, some of us have very fertile soil for good tissue health, and others have infertile soil with lots of weeds and nasty pathogens, simply by our bodies being too acidic, or in some cases, too alkaline. Pathogens can be looked upon as a naturally occurring organism out of its "proper" environment. The pathogen is invited to live in a foreign place by having the proper, (yet unhealthy for the body), conditions for its growth readily available. Nature dislikes a vacuum, so will fill the environment, (internal or external to the body,) with what it needs in a given terrain.

How do we move our body fluid and tissues into a more alkaline state for better immunity? How do we achieve better cellular regeneration abilities, lowered mucus levels, and lower inflammation levels? This has to do with diet and lifestyle choices for the most part. Modern science is currently, recognizing most diseases are related to deregulated inflammation processes in the body and virtually all degenerative disease is born in this inflammatory acidic state.

LIVER HEALTH

The liver function becomes more impaired with an increase in acid levels in the body fluid and tissues. Poor liver health can be experienced as high-stress levels, feeling short-tempered, being jaundiced, having portal vein hypertension, varicose veins, hemorrhoids, gallstones, bruising and bleeding, and loss of appetite. Having an overloaded liver can create a myriad of thinking, concentration, and sleeping problems as well. Most endocrine functions, which maintain hormone balance, depend not only on healthy pineal, pituitary, hypothalamus balance, but also on a healthy liver function.

Liver function is also damaged, or impaired by exposure to toxins, synthetic chemicals, such as non-steroidal anti-inflammation medications, most pharmaceutical drugs, parasites, fungal infections, pesticides, petroleum products, and cleaning products.

Even the shampoo, soaps and cosmetics a person uses end up being processed by the liver because our skin is a semi-permeable membrane, which allows for whatever products we use on our skin to enter our blood stream. This in turn, creates an extra burden on the liver.

It is so important to live within the concept—**"If you can't eat something, then don't be putting it on your body!"**

For many people, even over-exposure to chemicals in their toothpaste can be toxic. It is worth noting here that fluoride found in many types of toothpaste is toxic to the thyroid gland, located in the throat just above the sternum. Young Living has created toothpaste that utilizes essential oils. It naturally beneficial compounds while using no sodium laurel sulfates, which are toxic to the optic nerves, especially in children and unborn fetuses.

One of the liver's major functions in the body is known as conjugation. Conjugation occurs in two fundamental phases: one water-soluble and one oil-soluble. This conjugation process functions to make toxins in the body less dangerous. Toxic agents from an internal or external source need to be made safer to be passed out of the body. The body uses normal pathways of detoxification, which include skin, lungs, the large intestine, urinary tract, sinuses, and all mucus membranes, as well as the menstrual cycle in women. We will cover more detailed information on detoxification pathways in the **Appendix.**

Maybe you're wondering why acid and alkaline balancing of our bodies has not been studied in greater detail? For the most part, it is because the solution to this type of problem tends to be more nutritional in nature, rather than drug oriented. The real "cure" takes compliance with lifestyle changes that many people find foreign or challenging.

A more balanced or alkaline environment in the body can be brought about paying attention to what we take into our bodies, as well as the type of personal care products we use, along with our environment.

As we digest and burn the nutrition with our body's engine of vitality, some foods are high acid producers, and some foods are more alkaline. For instance, alfalfa and barley grass, uncooked raw or even dried vegetables have a very high alkaline action in the body. So do radishes, wheat grass, spinach, cucumbers, cayenne peppers, celery, and horseradish.

Young Living's NingXia Red also helps in bringing the body into Ph balance and acts as a natural anti-inflammatory.

In comparison, some foods are extremely acid-forming in the body. One of the very worst acidifying foods is pork. Vegetables bring the body into balance if a person has high Ph levels. Pork, beef, beer, chicken, veal, refined sugar (or white sugar), alcoholic liquor, white flour, and coffee are all acid forming. Sweetened or concentrated fruit juices are high in fructose corn syrup, and acid metabolites. Most soda pop is also an extremely acidic forming food since many soda pops have phosphoric acid added as a stabilizer.

Soda drinks with artificial sweeteners have ad extremely damaging effect on the endocrine system, far beyond disrupting the acid/alkaline balance of the consumer. This is due in part to the excite-toxin nature of artificial sweeteners on nerve and brain tissues, as well as endocrine tissues. These toxins disrupt the balance of the pituitary and pineal functions and trigger many food cravings, especially sweets.

Also, high fructose corn syrup is used in many commercial foods because it is inexpensive. It is linked to diabetes and blood sugar imbalances-- a virtual plague in America at this time. More and more Americans are classified as pre-diabetic due to dietary misinformation and junk food marketing and subsequent consumption beginning at an early age, sometimes by the parents prior to birth.

A change in pH balance creates acid and in most cases causes cravings for sweets, due to the need for more minerals in the body. We do not make minerals inside the body; we must find them in our diet, as well as be able to absorb them. Originally, humans found those minerals in their fruits and vegetables. Unfortunately, available junk foods tend to be mineral deficient and cause an array of health issues, since no amount of the wrong nutrients or anti-nutrients can make up for missing elements of nutrition, nor do the job of minerals. Whereas, if a person satisfies cravings by thinking like a caveman, going out to find fruit, a sweet nut, or a sweet vegetable, chances are those craving will be better satisfied. Also, fresh lemon or lemon oil and water can also help satisfy those cravings, as well as having an alkalizing effect on the body tissues. This may be why we like to drink lemonade. However, it is very important to take care not to use too much sweetener, or the lemons health benefits will be lost. Agave is a good sweetening agent, plus, it is very low on the glycemic index. This means it will not cause a spike in blood sugar like honey or sugar would.

ESSENTIAL OILS

It is interesting to note that an aspect of pure therapeutic grade essential oils is they have actions that are both molecular and energetic, and seem to be able to detoxify human cells in a remarkable way, similar to what a homeopathic remedy can do. The essential oils are created by photosynthesis in the action of plants transmitting sunlight, water, and minerals into nutrients and essential oils making Basil smell like what we think of as Basil or a lemon smell like a lemon. These aromatic components are often found to be the most bioactive aspect of the plant.

The energetic nature of essential oils and their life force also provides an interesting ability to balance emotional states. They have the ability to go directly into nervous system faster than any other method of intake and with no filters affecting the amygdale; a small almond sized glandular structure near the center of the brain having a relationship to how the body functions, during and after traumatic stress. This type of process is described, in detail, in numerous recent books and studies, my favorite being, "Releasing Emotional Patterns with Essential Oils, "by Dr. Carolyn Mein.

The ideal molecular qualities of pure essential oils properly distilled, is to retain the nature of their source, allowing transfer of oil molecules to a person, in a nutritional way, as well as vital essence of the plant then to be transferred to a person, in a vibrational way. Some scientific studies have shown that the way aromatic molecules smell to an individual has to more to do with vibrational rate (like the ringing of a bell) frequencies than the size, or shape of the molecule.

Aromatherapy is a bridge vibration of the plant kingdom; extending that bridge between the plant and animal kingdom including humans. Aromatherapy has a vibrating nature, a chemical nature, and emotional quality--all of which affect persons who receive it. Tests were conducted exposing individuals to molecules of similar shapes and sizes that had very dissimilar perceptions of smell. When the same tests were performed on molecules of similar vibrational frequencies, the tests showed that those molecules had a similar perception of a smell. So, in essence, it is the vibration of a molecule that gives it the recognizable aroma, not the shape or size.

Essential oils help reduce anxiety on many levels. Even when stress and anxiety are caused by trauma from years past; aromatherapy can help a person from being stuck in a flight or fight response, and therefore, lower the hormone imbalances, cortisol levels, and reduce internal acid build up in the body. Some health conditions are impossible to bring to balance or heal without addressing the underlying emotional blockages and unresolved emotional trauma. Often, **limiting beliefs** that have been programmed into someone since childhood no longer serve their original purpose, and, in fact, may be creating a dangerous and self-defeating set of thought patterns. Don't **believe everything you think.**

SYNTHETIC AROMATIC AIR FRESHENERS AND SYNTHETIC OILS

Most cheap air fresheners use synthetic oils and toxic chemicals. Some synthetic oils and synthetic enhancers are added to other aromatherapy oils, which are toxic and have constituents similar to insecticides, and endocrine disruptors. This process of making fake scents is known as "adulteration" when oils are promoted as being natural or pure essential oils, or in more recent industry language an "adjustment." Adulterated or adjusted oils are from various sources, which are not concerned with health and wellness of the end user and are usually significantly cheaper than the real thing. Therapeutic-grade oils are rare, due to the cost of growing, harvesting, and distilling the proper herbs and oils. Some adulterated components can be quite toxic, and, unfortunately, perfectly legal because essential oils are marketed and controlled similarly to cosmetics. If an essential oil used therapeutically, it is imperative to know and trust your source.

In France, a recent accounting of lavender growers showed that approximately 15 tons of true lavender oil was grown in a given year. Due to high market demand and chemical additive "adjustments," approximately 400 tons of oil was shipped and sold in that same year. Often Lavandin is sold as Lavender because of the similar smell and appearance. However, the actions are notably different, and one cannot be substituted for the other.

Make sure your oils are from a reputable source like Young Living Essential Oils. There are others that may be okay, but dollar for dollar there are few that match the quality or efficacy of Young Living Essential Oils. Also, when you buy from Young Living, you are purchasing years of highly documented scientific studies, and clinical experience that Young Living has funded. There is no substitute for getting this kind of university research regarding the efficacy of natural health and healing methods. Support this continuing effort in researching nature's gifts to mankind.

Andrea's visit--September 14, 2005:

During the initial visit with Andrea, I determined some of her meridians were out of balance. The points in her body and corresponding meridians that were out of balance included: her lungs, large intestines, circulation, allergies, reactivity (immune system), triple warmer, heart, pancreas, gall bladder, bladder, and cartilage (tissue between joints) lower body. This was just after Andrea's second miscarriage.

During the intake, Andrea had symptoms of a headache, exhaustion, and dehydration. She then stated she was working on a computer eight hours a day. Computers usually emit various forms of perverse energy, so I suggested a screen protector to minimize this energy. She had a history of drinking sodas and tea beverages containing the sweetener Aspartame/NutraSweet, which is not only an excitotoxin, but has a stimulating and addictive nature to it. This category of artificial sweeteners is linked to some health issues, including obesity and pituitary imbalance, anxiety, depression, and attention deficit disorders. She also had a history of allergies; she was given over 100 shots for two years. She went on to say she was having a yeast infection at least once a year, and family history of cervical cancer.

My recommendation at this time was a female tonic. A bottle of the xenobiotic homeopathic remedy to dispel toxic, "food additives," and a reminder to avoid exposures to electronic devices, such as cathode ray screens, computer screens, and strong electromagnetic fields. I also reminded her to get a screen protector and to avoid all artificial sweeteners. The importance of reading labels and being educated about the varied names for these toxins is very important.

Andrea's, visit--October 13, 2005:

During the intake for this month, Andrea was feeling better. She mentioned doing a liver cleanse in January 2005, and she thought this time she was pregnant. Her symptoms were a yeast infection and sneezing a lot like a cold.

For this visit, my recommendation was for Andrea to continue using the female tonic, an anti-stress remedy, and the NingXia Red, a fortifying juice from

Young Living Essential Oils. Then each day she doubled the dosage for about four days to rid her body of the yeast infection. I encouraged her to use the hormonal creams: Progessence and Prenelone, as recommended by Deanna Romero, P.A.

Aromatherapy oils were recommended to treat her stress. They included White Angelica and Abundance, with the appropriate affirmations, and alarm as suggested in the book, "Releasing Emotional Patterns with Essential Oils," by Dr. Carolyn Mein.

Andrea's visit--November 22, 2005:

The intake for this month was Andrea experiencing a lack of sleep. She did the mermaid wrap and had a previous herbal wrap in June of 2005. Andrea felt her menstrual cycle was improving because her period went from three days to four days. Her meridians were improving: lungs balanced, immune system, tissue degeneration was high—68, but dropped to 40. Her liver meridian was low but getting higher.

I discussed with Andrea the importance of R.E.M. sleep. A woman wanting to achieve a successful pregnancy should get to sleep before midnight. The body needs sleep to balance hormone levels and a consistent sleep pattern of going to bed no later than 10:30 p.m. is strongly encouraged.

HORMONES AND EXCITOTOXINS

Our bodies produce hormones constantly, and during the early morning, the hormone called Cortisol is produced to counter balance the human growth hormone – HGH. Cortisol is produced after the body produces adrenaline, such as in a fight or flight response. During our sleep cycles, especially early in the night, the body produces the human HGH. This master hormone aids in vitality and tissue rejuvenation, and is imperative for a healthy pregnancy, as well as keeping us youthful in appearance and a metabolism.

Synthetic sweeteners are classified as Excitotoxins: aspartame, acesulfame, phenylalanine, artificial colors or flavorings-all cause the Cortisol level to go higher. This often causes tissue damage and rapid aging, rather than regenerating cellular tissues, as with normal healthy hormone balances. Excitotoxins also imbalance the pituitary and pineal glands in ways that keep an individual from being able to access their intuitive qualities, as well as inhibit the production of HGH which is a master hormone required to regenerate tissue, promote healing, and keep you looking YOUNG! On top of that, these toxins are addictive!

Studies in Wisconsin have shown that children in grade school and high school often cannot focus, or learn properly, due to junk food consumption. Schools are beginning to catch on, by banning junk food vending machines that have become popular cash cows for schools over the last twenty years.

I once met a woman who was making her living by putting vending units in schools that sold sugarless gum loaded with artificial sweeteners. She, herself, had become so addicted to the sweeteners that she was constantly on the verge of having an anxiety panic attack. During every attack, I witnessed her reaching for more of the excitotoxic gum. She did not want to hear the truth about what she was doing to herself.

And at one time, aspartame was listed by the Pentagon as a potential biological weapon. Nazi and chemical warfare themes are a recurring part of aspartame trail. An interesting fact that some of the parent companies that produces these excitotoxins are also parent companies of corporations that want to try to sell synthetic drugs for depression and anxiety, one creating the need for the other.

Recent studies indicate artificial sweeteners cause obesity and unhealthy food cravings, usually sugar or other sweets. When we eat sugar frequently, we create stress to many of our organ systems, lower our immunity, imbalance our blood sugar, take in empty calories that lead to deficiencies in other nutrients, especially minerals. When we eat sugar laden foods, a fungus can rapidly grow in our bodies. Sugar is the perfect food for fungal growth. Fungal infections can be low grade, last for years undetected, and cause immune system stress, chronic fatigue, swelling in many tissues, especially the spleen, as well as contribute to many forms of cancer, and tumors.

CONSTITUTIONAL HOMEOPATHY
After working with Andrea, I considered whether a constitutional homeopathic remedy would be applicable. It is usually the best form of treatment, especially considering

that it could greatly improve the health of any offspring for future generations to come. Constitutional homeopathy treats the total person; all aspects of a person's life, health, vitality, and wellness. It is considered to be the highest and truest form of homeopathic treatment. As with any treatment plan, it is also important to reduce obstacles that stand in the way of a person's health, and that includes diet, lifestyle, and toxic and perverse energy exposure.

Homeopathy helps overcome obstacles by bringing the body into wholeness. As previously discussed, single type remedies are used for classical style treatment and there about 4000 types. Choosing the correct remedy and potency is the key.

OBSTACLES TO THE CURE
In conclusion, obstacles to the cure can be external influences, such as being exposed to a video or computer terminal. The electrical, magnetic radiation signal is usually not compatible with human or other biological energy. Recent studies are showing that repeated cell phone exposure causes cellular mutation and imbalances, and can possible cause brain tumor in younger frequent users. Every day, we see people with a phone tied to their head, and becoming in appearance, a person that half human, half robot. A constant long-term level of electromagnetic radiation will cause cellular degeneration of numerous types. Pregnant women should avoid exposures to all forms of perverse energy.

Micro-waved foods are also a common cause of problems. It has been shown that microwaves cause molecular changes in food that allow some proteins to become plastics and indigestible, as well as reduce available nutrients such as enzymes. **Microwaves are not biocompatible** *to living organisms. I have seen cases of emotional imbalances in sensitive people caused by using microwaves to heat water--an element key to human life, which makes up around 80 percent of our body weight.*

Obstacles to cure can be an addiction to diet soda drinks with artificial sweeteners, or any number of other problem causing habits. It can also be an addiction to other stimulants, so it is useful to analyze how much caffeine we are drinking, as well as a look at the use of nearly any substance on a regular basis. Too many of these various ingredients that act as stimulants or depressants can deprive our bodies of nutrients by burning up large amounts of some nutrients and creating an excess of others. The regular use of synthetic drugs and cosmetics can also be a large obstacle to curing.

Our lifestyles in this modern world can be obstacles themselves. For example: an old knee injury that causes inflammation of cartilage tissue can be worsened by being exposed on a day to day basis to excess sugar from to eating two and three candy bars a day, accompanied by artificially sweetened or colored beverages. These are not the foods nature intended us to eat. Staying up late into the night watching extensive TV, working on a computer, or reading a book can cause the flight or fight syndrome, raising levels of the hormone Cortisol. In many cases, we are exercising less, resting less, and facing more stress in our daily lives. Is it worth the damage these poor habits cause on our health?

*Obstacles to cure can also be **limiting belief** about any number of things that create a blockage of flow, and potentially a lack of success. The obstacles can occur in areas such as relationships, health issues, or right livelihood. Simply being in a constant state of negativity, or being a subject of abuse, can also be obstacles to a fully developed and healthy life.*

ANDREA'S SUMMARY

After working with Carl for four months, in one month's time my hair grew two inches. Normally, my hair grows an inch every two months. Carl suggested doing another cleanse for the intestines. After completing this cleansing, my intestines whistled. I could feel air flowing in and out of my anal. My body was completely cleaned out. My readings on all organs were between 45 and 55. I was finally feeling very healthy! So, when my buttocks whistled, this was a sign. It was time. But, also consider before you become pregnant, the health of your partner. In the next chapter, Carl discusses Men's health.

MEN'S HEALTH BY CARL JANICEK

One issue I have noted in dealing with male health issues is the reticence of a great number of men to broach the subject at all. It seems the common perception or "group think" going through the minds of our male population is that if there is a problem with conception or the baby's health, then it surely must be the woman's fault.

It is almost as though there is a great fear among men regarding their sexual prowess and their genetic legacy. Why else would men be so easily hypnotized by the common advertising of "male enhancement" products sold in magazines and television or the libido stimulators that pharmaceutical companies sell in great quantities?

Maslow's hierarchy of needs states that a satisfied need is not a motivator....

Most men don't seem to know good nutrition and regular exercise have the same libido enhancing effects as popular fad synthetic enhancers! This is a best-kept secret in our society. Is it possible men who lack natural libido (sex drive) simply aren't fit (according to nature) to reproduce? Is it possible many of today's children with genetic flaws would not exist if men who are not healthy did not reproduce? I know this is controversial thinking, but ultimately these questions will be answered by the laws of nature.

It is true the major responsibility of carrying the fetus to full term, resides with the mother and her ability to eat nutritious meals, avoid high-stress levels, and toxic exposures. Such toxic exposures include, but are not limited to artificial sweeteners, flavorings, coloring, tobacco, soda pop, Tran's fat (preserved fats) and micro-waved foods. After the birth of the baby, there is no substitute for breast feeding along with a home environment free from as many artificial and toxic exposures as possible.

There is responsibility on the part of the father to reinforce and support the mother during her nine months of the life-giving process. His health must be in top condition prior to conception. This requires both mental and physical functioning at the highest levels, to prepare his "seed" to be his legacy for the future generations of his family.

There are considerable pressures in our current work world for men to be "macho," which push them to "tough it out" regardless of any hazards. Far too many men are caught up in this trap. It is the false pretension to admire productivity and a "macho" image over and above the quality of seed we men should contribute to the future legacy of our family and our world. Modern medicine might call it genetic mutation, or have some other rationale, but we men have far more control over these issues than we are being told. To have a healthy baby then healthy sperm is an absolute necessity.

Overall, steps necessary to balance a man's body are similar to those needed to balance a woman's body. Regardless of what our current culture says, the difference between a man's body and a woman's body at the cellular level are amazingly similar. There may be slight variations in nutrient needs between men and women. All in all the need for basically clean air and water, essential fatty acids, minerals, and nutrients are largely the same.

One factor in men's health that has been recognized by modern science is exposure to certain industrial chemicals such as paints, plastics, insecticides, heavy metals, (such as those found in some dental materials,) can greatly affect a man's sexual health, including libido and sperm count. Again, to have a healthy baby then healthy sperm is an absolute necessity. A man's body will not be able to produce healthy sperm if he lacks proper nutrition, carries excess residual compounds from stress, or if he carries excess toxic exposures from a variety of pollutants. Men's bodies require slightly more nutrients, such as zinc and vitamin E than a woman's body. Ultimately, each nutrient needs are determined more by their genetic makeup and lifestyle choices than by gender.

In these modern times the value of our seed, once held sacred by our ancestors, has been lost, forgotten, or deliberately buried to pursue wealth, status, and power. This was caused by the hypnotic illusion of our culture created by consumerism and corporations. This illusion lacks soul, and it values nothing other than financial gain. Unfortunately, this wealth gathering is a hollow victory, and it lacks the gift of health which we should bequeath to our children and their children to follow. Wealth is a great gift--far better than poverty--on so many levels. However, wealth without true health is greatly diminished in its value. Wealth is truly best when experienced together with good health.

"A woman goes to the see the doctor in her car; a man goes in an ambulance!"

Seeing a homeopath is not restricted to just women. However, generally women have habits reinforced by our cultural biases to take better care of their selves. If consumers of the modern medical establishment do not get answers on why they do not feel well, it is a good time for them to see an alternative type of practitioner.

Modern commercialized medicine, particularly in America, is prone to crisis management rather than giving a lot of attention to the basic foundation of good health provided by proper nutrition. It is said by many people that in America today we have sick care, but not healthcare.

Much of modern medicine is influenced by pharmaceutical companies that have a vested interest in their products being prescribed by physicians. One of the large factors creating inefficiency in American healthcare is that insurance companies determine how, when, and if a provider will be paid. These corporations are protected by faulty legislation that guards them against antitrust regulations--a terrible mistake. Insurers are profiting from the denial of some care and limiting other types of care. This creates conflicts between the need for preventative care, good holistic health education, and the system that is currently in place. America spends 16 percent of its gross domestic product (GDP) on healthcare, and currently "the industry" is saying in the next few years these costs may go as high as 20 to 24 percent of our GDP. America only ranks of 37th in the world for quality of health care, as determined by the World Health Organization. This organization takes into consideration infant mortality, longevity, as well as the availability and cost of care.

Many other countries spend far less on health care than Americans, yet receive far better care. For example:

France spends approximately 11 percent of its Gross Domestic Product (GDP) on health care, yet this country is ranked the number one country in health care provision.

England spends approximately eight percent of its GDP on healthcare, but this modern country is ranked at number 18.

Steps for balancing a man's body are similar to balancing a woman's body. Regardless of what our current culture says, the difference between a man's body and a woman's body is at the cellular level, which is amazingly similar. There might be slight variations in nutrient needs between men and women. All in all, the basic needs for good air and water, essential fatty acids, minerals, and other nutrients and largely the same for both men and women.

CLEANSING THE BODY

Cleansing the male body is carried out in much the same way as for cleansing the female body, but with males there is a need for more exercise to cause the body to sweat. Men do not have a menstrual cycle. Therefore, detoxification pathways available to women are not available to men.

Men's use of anti-nutrients, including junk food, recreational drugs, or pharmaceuticals can take longer to clear from a man's body than a woman's body. For this reason, the mental, physical and emotional health of the man, as well as his diet, must be in harmony with the goal of having a healthy child.

Men are proud of their children, as evidenced by the glow on a new father's face. It would be wise counsel to start that glow, a year before conception. Men's immune systems are partially regulated by their blood type, so if a man is willing to study his blood type, his proper nutritional needs, along with compatible foods, then the process to become healthier is a lot cheaper.

Men's jobs, careers, and work environment are often less healthy than those of women's. There is a certain "macho" aura of having a dirty job or being able to handle a high-stress executive position, but all in all men's health suffers from these types of scenarios. Instead, men need to take responsibility to do their "personal cleanse," improve their dietary habits, and to avoid bad lifestyle choices, such as drugs and alcohol. Ultimately, men are to handle their state of health. For most men, diet, exercise, and meditation may be sore subjects. However, for these same men, the benefits of good health can be dramatically improved when they take this subject seriously and focus on these areas.

There are a number of cleansing techniques and processes available including the Master Cleanse, as described by Stanley Burroughs in his book, "The Master Cleanser" and a much easier "5 Day Cleanse," produced by Young Living Essential Oils. Please talk to a licensed professional for updated product.

MERIDIAN BASED ASSESSMENT...

When a person comes into my office for help, usually they've seen several healthcare practitioners, yet their health problems have not been resolved. They do not have the solution for the challenges to their health. As a consultant, I work to resolve these challenges in a way compatible to their philosophies of life. Often I help them find solutions that aren't available through the current structure of Western Medicine.

People come in for initial screening and evaluation through the use of a meridian stress assessment. This stress assessment has been around for thousands of years. Traditionally, Chinese medicine used meridian assessment by studying pulses at different positions on the wrist, observing the person's general condition of a person. They also studied alarm points on the body that have associations with specific meridian energy flows (chi or life force). These meridian energy flows are analogous in form. Through this process of assessment, it is possible to gain insights into overall health, vitality, and stress affecting the person.

It is possible to gain insight into meridians, alarm points, and stress levels by using test equipment that measures galvanic skin responses and Kinesiology. While modern medicine does not tend to use these types of tests, similar tests are practiced, that include taking a person's temperature, noting their pulse and respiration, measuring brain waves with an EEG, and measuring heart rhythms and electrical activity using an EKG. Criminologists use galvanic skin response testing, in conjunction with heart rate and respiration to determine if a subject displays abnormal stress, such as with the use of a lie detector. So, while modern medicine is willing to use many electro-measurement devices, there seems to be a perceptual deficiency in modern medicine in the area of the meridian stress assessment. Possibly this is due to the influence drug companies have over medical education. All in all, these instruments and methodologies are measuring the response to stimuli by the body.

The word "electrical" was coined by an English physician named William Gilbert. Around the year 1600, he established the difference between electricity and magnetism. Then close to the year 1830, a professor of physics, Carlo Matteucci, showed that electrical current is generated by injured tissues. Later Dr. Frances described the relief of dental pain by the use of electricity, and in 1631 he performed tooth extractions using "Galvanism." He was then granted a patent on May 26, 1858. During those times, electrical rate, and these results were confirmed in the University College Hospital in London, England.

Around the year 1900 in the United States, high government officials were often corrupted by large corporate interests. Much like today, this included stock market manipulations, allowing contaminated or imbalanced beef to be shipped to soldiers in far off wars, and medicine was offered to cure every ailment known to man. This problem, accompanied by a long a lack of standards, medical education, along with poor practices, produced situations easily manipulated by pharmaceutical interests. Even today insurance companies are too often involved in supporting political and publicity campaigns that further their profits. Sometimes these companies even go to the point where they create and fund "non-profit" and "public interest" groups that further the distribution of doubt and create grey information to keep the public confused. So long as corporate interests are valued by the government above the interests of the individual, we will continue to pay the price of ignorance.

There are other interests hoping to sell methodologies to Americans in search of better health or cures. However, they have to pass through the current flawed system of approval, so rarely do any actual cures make it to the market due to many special interests that influence the political and legal environment.

A German doctor developed an electronic testing device capable of finding acupuncture points in the early 1950's. Dr. Voll studied this procedure passionately. As a result, he was able to identify the correlation between diseases, acupuncture points, and their resistance. In his research, he amassed a great deal of information that showed the accuracy of his methods and discoveries. All in all, using an experienced practitioner who is properly trained in traditional Chinese Medicine, as well as in Galvanic skin response measurement that uses proper equipment, a great deal of insight can be gained in cases that may not be resolved by any other method. Meridian stress tests are performed around the world using instruments that are manufactured in Germany, Japan, China, France, Denmark, Russia, and the United States. Many double-blind studies have been used to determine the validity of the concept.

PRACTITIONER'S NOTE:

When I am seeing a new client, I use concepts of meridians and their balance to help me get an overview of the case, as well as to be able to validate and offer potential remedial actions. After I have tested a subject to find stressed or blocked meridians, it is of great importance to inquire further about the client's condition, especially about their exposure to specific toxins. It is also important to gather the client's lifestyle information and get specifics of his/her dietary habits. In this manner, the client is the final determinant as to whether my assessment of the meridians correlates with their health and personal experience.

Once correlations are found for a given person, recommended treatments or protocols that increase the subject's overall health and wellness by reducing stress to the meridians are then implemented. One of the great values of this test method is that regardless how many books I have read, or how many studies I have undertaken, the recommendations made by the use of meridian assessments are unique to the individual being studied at that moment in time. This conclusion is based on experiences with clients in my office. This has proved to be true whether I am using a constitutional type of homeopathic remedy based on their totality of symptoms or upon a shallower approach, using reductionistic principles.

This methodology, while not perfect for all aspects of a case, allows for a treatment plan and therapies to be totally and uniquely attuned to the client's vital force in that specific moment.

It is also interesting to note while there is a plethora of companies selling nutritional products and supplements from A to Z. Many of these companies succumb to the idea that cheaper is better. Therefore, they use the cheapest ingredients available to them. Sometimes these companies end up buying raw components of unknown quality just to meet a price point.

One of the reasons I believe in using products from Young Living, as well as some other manufacturers of high-quality nutrition, essential oils, and homeopathy is these products tend to test well with high positive outcomes, as seen consistently in clients coming into my office.

SOUL SEARCHING AND ETHICAL CONSIDERATIONS OF MIDLIFE CHILD BEARING

Many people might consider a lack of human reproductive fertility a form of natural selection. There is also the possibility this is a motivating path to raise awareness in certain industrialized populations that are mainly responsible for the contamination of the earth's precious soil, water and air—major elements of our habitat. This is a critical, yet simple lesson for humanity to learn. We cannot continue to act in an ignorant or denial-based manner concerning our waste production resulting in biosphere destruction. Furthermore, we cannot continue to accept the idea that we can continue to throw things away. Instead, we must learn to recycle our used things back to nature. Our habitat, the earth's biosphere, is a circulating, closed system in which we play a major role by our choices. We must include our population density.

In most industrialized cultures, there are many factors that have contributed to the self- destructive manner in which humans are currently living. As the density of population goes up, quality of life goes down. A looming possibility is humans may either create or avoid the next mass extinction on earth by our very attitudes, idea, and emotions towards each other, our children, and our planet. The earth may have already reached its critical capacity for human consumer behavior.

One question this raises is whether child bearing past the ideal years of normal healthy reproduction will have a weakening or strengthening outcome for the human race and genetic lines? Statistics shows that parenting after the age of 40 has much greater risks for the mother and child, as well as on the health of our social systems. This is due in part to the much higher possibility of birth defects, as well as problems older parents have with learning and behavioral issues on the part of their children.

On occasion, there news articles and headlines written about first-time mothers conceiving children in their late 40's, early 50's, and even 60's. It's obvious these parents may not be up to the task of rearing children when they complain about how they are tired much of the time and easily depressed. Also, they don't know how to get their daily routines back to "normal."

Well, guess what? These parents may have not done the math, or considered the fact that in our current world rearing a young child takes considerable time, energy, and other resources, including large financial commitments in order to bring their child, even a healthy one, into adulthood.

There is the possible advantage older parents will have better economic resources and more table relationships, which can be beneficial to their offspring on many levels. There is also the risk relationships older parents form with their children may never be the same as those younger parents have with their children, since differences in age may classify these parents as "too old" to understand or participate in the child's development at certain crucial times in his or her young life.

There is also a common period in the upbringing of any child, known as puberty, which is challenging to any parent. Puberty can last for a great portion of the teen years, and it is questionable whether anyone in their 60's or 70's would choose to be in the midst of teen adventures and misadventures for 24 hours a day, 7 days a week. Just this type of scenario may be part of the consequence of having a child later in life.

I have a sister-in-law who has worked as a nurse in the maternity wards of major hospitals. She has always seen a flow of babies born to teenage mothers, who are largely unprepared to take on the responsibility of childrearing. She reports that another disturbing trend is "late in life" mothers, sometimes even in their 50's, giving birth to babies who are often not as vital as babies born by younger mothers. These babies then end up with a multitude of complications themselves. Sometimes these disabilities are so bad; their parents must hire help just to get through each day.

Usually, it does not take a high skill level to have a baby. However, it does take skill, education, and a vast amount of caring, patience, and parenting time to raise a child to become a healthy adult. A great number of infertility issues may be a normal, natural response to a wide range of environmental factors. Some of these may be caused by an already over-populated world with humans being the largest factor in the destruction of our biosphere and habitat. If you are considering having a child in your midlife, then there is a multitude of complex factors to examine carefully and rationally according to your life situation. Of course, this decision is often based on the underlying emotional needs of the parents, rather than on the reality of their situation, or upon rational behavior.

THE GORILLA IN THE ROOM--OVER POPULATION ISSUES

Over population of any species is a condition where the number of the organism exceeds the carrying capacity of its habitat. **Overpopulation refers to a condition in which population density enlarges to a limit that provokes deterioration of the environment** *along with a remarkable decline in the quality of life, which may lead to the collapse of that population.*

Every ten years, almost one billion human inhabitants are added to the world's population. If the world's population continues to grow at an average of three children per couple, the global population for 2050 will be 10.5 billion inhabitants, of whom 7.7 billion will suffer from extreme poverty, lack of fresh water, hunger, illnesses, and other types of problems.

Mechanisms automatically activated in nature when a population grows to its extremes do exist. These ordinary mechanisms are sequentially put into action, as soon as the populations break the limits their habitats can sustain. Some of these mechanisms for humans include wars, an increase of crime, hunger, epidemics, emergent and re-emergent illnesses, genetic degradation, and so forth.

ECONOMIC CONSIDERATIONS

Having a child is a far greater financial responsibility than having a pet, which in many cases is surprisingly expensive, too. As a parent, you are responsible your health and well-being, but also the care, feeding, clothing, and education of your child. This should be obvious to people who consider childbearing, yet it appears this is often a "second thought" after the child is born. A healthy infant can cost relatively little for the first few months, yet overall costs will steadily climb for the next 21 years, culminating in the expense of higher education. Recent calculations show that raising a healthy child costs approximately $200,000 in the first 20 years.

These challenging economic times are a stress factor for many individuals. Breadwinners for families can tell you they feel more financial uncertainty than ever before. Will both parents find themselves needing to work full-time with the possibility of having to have some paid or unpaid surrogate raising their child? Is this what you would choose for your child? Is a daycare center the best answer for child rearing? During the first 18 years of a child's life, there is no real substitute for Mom or Dad.

If you are not able to support your offspring emotionally, as well as financially, until they are adults--sometimes well into adulthood, the burden may end up being passed on to other members of your family. In a dire scenario, they may end being taken care of by some form of social services. What happens to a child born with exceptional difficulties and needs? An unhealthy child can become such a huge burden emotionally and financially that families end up breaking apart and declaring bankruptcy. Do you and your mate have risk factors that could cause your child to have more than average health issues? How is your current state of health and vitality? Are you in the best of shape? Currently, over 50 percent of all bankruptcies in America today are due to medical costs. These are some of the questions couples should ponder before taking the big step into parenthood.

RETIREMENT

When are you planning or hoping to retire? Do you think you have saved enough to have a reasonable standard of living when you do retire? Do you plan to have the expenses associated with raising a child during your retirement? Do you plan to work into your 70's to support your child? Do you plan to have government taxpayer-funded programs support you in retirement, such as Social Security, which, in fact, may no longer exist? These are sometimes difficult questions to ask. However, not asking them may lead to much greater difficulties, more stress, and even damage to your health during the later part of your life. Otherwise, this might be a time when you would choose to enjoy much more freedom and independence.

If you have any questions or doubts regarding these types of issues, then it would be wise to seek independent professional counseling for such a large life path decision and life change as that which would be brought on by the birth of a child in your later years. I would recommend that you do not seek this type of decision-making counsel from anyone associated with a fertility clinic or any clinic having a financially vested interest in the outcome you choose. Today, babies are a very big business with some fertility specialists earning millions of dollars a year, and they have strong financial reasons to encourage people to use their services. At this time, the ethics held by practitioners in this professional specialty are questionable.

"THIRD TIME IS A CHARM:" BEGINNING OF A SUCCESSFUL PREGNANCY:

FIRST TRIMESTER:
MONTH 1:

In January 2006, I recall my chiropractic treatment and a talk with Dr. Maxfield, she asked, "Are you pregnant?" I said, "No." She went on to explain that it's possible my ovulation cycle had changed. She showed me that I could purchase ovulation kits for as little as one dollar and directed me to places where I could purchase them. Also, just prior to my conversation with Dr. Maxfield, I spoke with a nurse from my own doctor's office. The nurse told me that when a woman knows she's ovulating, her and her partner should have sexual intercourse on the day of ovulation and the day after. In my case, I purchased my kit, and I used it to identify my menstrual cycle had changed in three months, from a nine-day cycle to a seven-day cycle.

> **TIPS:** I suggest purchasing ovulation kits to determine when ovulation occurs. Then, when the test is positive for ovulation, have intercourse the day of ovulation and the day after. The nurse I spoke with told me that this increases chances of fertilization and pregnancy by maximizing the amount of available sperm to penetrate the egg.
>
> In her book, "Taking Charge of your Fertility," author Toni Weschler says, "As discussed in the preceding chapter, it is imperative couples should not use artificial lubricants or saliva, since these can actually kill sperm" p. 185.

Also, this is just my theory; having sex at night increased my chance of conception and resulted in pregnancy. I took a mere bathroom break, went to sleep, and then bathed the following morning.

During this time, I continued taking the natural supplements from Young Living as recommended by Carl Janicek. The supplements included the following Young Living products:

Hers (multi-vitamin),
Vitamin C
Ninja Red Juice
Super-Cal
Prenelone
Progessence

I also used the following two items are not manufactured by Young Living: Socar's Folic Acid and Carlson's Super Omega-3 Fish oil. Please know some of the product has been upgraded, so consult a licensed professional about your vitamins.

I took the advice given to me by my friend and Physician's Assistant, Deanna Romero, Dr.

Maxfield and Carl Janicek on improving my nutrition. I started eating foods that were more fortifying such as organic, raw fruits and vegetables. I reduced my consumption of foods that were frozen, canned or cooked in the microwave unless they were organic products. Like most of us, I am by no means perfect about eating and maintaining a healthy diet. I ate minimal servings of junk food, and limited consumption of this type food to special occasions such as my sister-in-law's 40th birthday celebration. Every four months I allowed myself to splurge on fast food, like French fries, or Chipotle. Then two times a month, I'd go to the grocery store to purchase a loaf of fresh baked or organic bread. This diet change was initially implemented four months prior to my pregnancy. I don't always eat healthy, but I strive for a well-balanced diet.

TIP: To purchase products from Young Living, check their website at youngliving.com or call their number at 1-800-371-3515. Please mention this book.

The supplements Carl recommended are mainly made from all-natural ingredients. The spices, herbs, antioxidants, and other ingredients can be found, growing naturally in our earth's environment. The way I understand this is my ancient indigenous ancestors would send a woman out into the desert, the plains, or the mountains for several days and observe whether or not she survived. If she lived, she was honored as the medicine woman or healer of the tribe. In Spanish, she is known as the "Curandera." They ate what nature provided and survived. As you know, in modern time, the ingredients are compressed, liquefied for consumption and made into tablets or capsules. I threw away the vast majority of the other synthetic supplements because, in my opinion, these supplements aren't natural.

Now, consider this about my sister-in-law who went to a fertility specialist. What supplements did her doctor prescribe, and how did this advice compare to my supplements? She said her specialist prescribed Vitamin C and additional antioxidants. I thought funny, Carl suggested the same thing. The Ninja Red manufactured by Young Living contains the powerful antioxidants: Ningxia wolfberry, blueberry, pomegranate, apricot, raspberry, grape, organic blend of blue agave, lemon, and orange. I hear claims about how a single antioxidant can help your body. Not! In my opinion try multiple antioxidants.

Something to consider, I thought to myself, "In 20 years will my child be able to eat antioxidants? Will antioxidants still be plentiful? Will two out of three people in the United States die from Cancer? Is the lack of organic antioxidants, spices, and herbs killing us? If we continue this path, our society dies out like those in the movie, *"Children of Men."* a plot where humans can no longer reproduce?" Have you heard that thousands upon thousands of bees are dying?

As a future mom, I realized a scenario like *"Children of Men"*, could occur. But I knew it was necessary to balance my body and continue to see Dr. Maxfield, to see Carl, and continue with my supplements. Another week went by, yet another week went by, and then I could smell burnt popcorn twenty-five feet away. Oh, then came the nausea, but I was fortunate because I never saw the porcelain God!

MONTH 2:

Oh no--it happened again--I am getting so stressed out at work. I thought to myself, "No one is helping me! Would I lose my baby? Dear God, not again please! I can't take the stress!" The stress and hormones were like a volcanic eruption within me. I was abrupt with customers all day long, and I couldn't control my reactions. Another day went by, and it happened again. Two days prior to this meltdown, I informed the management of my pregnancy. I was scared to tell them because I was fearful of retaliation.

In the book entitled, *"What To Expect When You're Expecting,"* by Heidi Murkoff, Arlene Eisenberg and Sandee Hathaway, B.S.N. says, "To expect emotional instability comparable to premenstrual syndrome, (probably more pronounced), which may include irritability, mood swings, irrationality and weepiness", page 135; 2002 edition.

After my meltdowns at work, I had my blood drawn. The nurse called a day later to tell me, "Your hormones levels are good. Schedule an ultrasound and come in for your first checkup." I then told her I had already scheduled the ultrasound for the following week.

The following week I was terminated from my place of employment. My ultrasound was good. After viewing the ultrasound picture, my uncle-in-law called his future niece, larva. My precious larva, "Aly," had a heartbeat of 180n beats per minute. She was normal in size, and she didn't appear to be a circular blob. Yes, the ultrasound showed a head and a body!

Note: Every day, I continually applied the hormone creams Progessence, (like progesterone), and Prenelone, plus I took natural supplements from Young Living: Master Hers multi-vitamin, Vitamin C, Ninja Red juice, Super-Cal, along with the following two items not manufactured by Young Living but made by Socar's Folic

Acid and Carlson's Super Omega-3 Fish Oil. As mentioned in month 1, I continued to try and eat a healthier diet. The supplements helped me maintain my healthy pregnancy. Please talk to licensed professionals for supplement recommendations.

MONTH 3:

Ah, home and relaxation, just what I needed! At last, I was getting more sleep. When I worked, I would go to sleep at eight p.m., and then wake up at five a.m., so I always felt exhausted. But as soon as I could stay home, full time, I averaged textbook sleep of about 10 to 12 hours a day.

Now, the second ultrasound was excellent. I was elated and as soon as I left the office, I started crying tears of joy. Finally! I felt bad about losing my job, but my friends, acquaintances and family all told me, "I was right where I needed to be-- at home resting and not risking another miscarriage." At this time, I reduced my exercise from using the treadmill 15 minutes three times a week to a 15-minute walk around the park, just two to three times a week. I wanted to make certain that I wouldn't miscarry.

After my first monthly check up, the nurse told me to schedule my next appointment with the doctor and this was the same nurse whom I had seen in the past. This nurse has the unfortunate job of telling patients when they are about to miscarry. She was there for the first miscarriage and the second miscarriage. So this time, she was happy for my husband and me.

Note: Every day, I continue to apply the hormone cream Progessence and take natural supplements from Young Living: Master Hers Multivitamin, Vitamin C, Ninja Red juice, Super-Cal, and the following two items not manufactured by Young Living, which are Socar's Folic Acid and Carlson Super Omega-3 Fish Oil. As mentioned in month 1, I continued to eat a healthier diet. Please talk to licensed professionals for supplement recommendations.

SECOND TRIMESTER

MONTH 4:

I had my checkup, and my doctor-is was ecstatic, as was I. It was hard to believe. But, it was time. I wouldn't give up. I just kept thinking positive thoughts about how beautiful our baby would be. Even if I did get a little anxious, I just kept thinking positive affirmations that my baby was coming, and I would not be denied the miracle of having my child.

I started experiencing constipation. And I am not a big advocate of man-made laxatives. I prefer to use a more natural laxative, my friend and my P.J. - Prune Juice not from concentrate. Deanna told me, "Andrea, drink the juices that aren't high in sugar. Purchase juices labeled "not from concentrate"." I verified with the doctor and asked," Is it ok to drink a quarter cup of P.J. every day?" She confirmed, "Yes, it is ok to drink a quarter cup each day." Also, consider there are alternative herbal laxatives and teas that help relieve constipation.

Note: Every day, I continually apply the hormone cream Progessence and take natural supplements from Young Living: Master Hers multivitamin, Vitamin C, Ninja Red juice, Super-Cal, the following items are not manufactured by Young Living and made by Socar's Folic Acid and Carlson's Super Omega-3 Fish Oil. As mentioned in month 1, I continued to try and eat a healthier diet. Please speak to a licensed, trained professional for updated recommendations for supplements.

MONTH 5:

She kicked me! Yeah! The Sciatic nerve, which is located in the back area, was causing me grief! Ouch! I scheduled a chiropractic adjustment. Dr. Maxfield explained that when the baby lies on one side of the uterus for a prolonged period, the opposite side will start aching.

During this time, I didn't notice a decrease in urination. There was no decrease in nausea. Now, my appetite did increase.

And Deanna would tell me, "Andrea, stay away from white flour and white sugar because you can give your baby gestational diabetes." However, again as I mentioned earlier in this book, I didn't eat a perfect, perfect diet. Every day, I ate chocolate Haagen Daz ice cream. I'd bake natural pork chops at least once a week for dinner accompanied by organic canned green beans. Being Mexican-American, I craved once a month smothered tamales covered in green chili, lettuce, tomato and cheese from Chubby's off of 38th Avenue in Denver. So, after sleeping 12 hours, I'd call ahead for my lunch order and then pick it up.

This month, we were in Minnesota, and on one of our vacation days we took a family photo. It was two p.m. and, I had no tolerance for the sun. I started feeling weak, faint, dehydrated, and I had just finished a bottle of water. Unfortunately, while I was there, the mosquitoes devoured my blood. All summer long, I couldn't go anywhere in Colorado and Minnesota because the love affair with mosquitoes.

Note: Every day, I continually applied the hormone cream Progessence and took natural supplements from Young Living: Master Hers multivitamin, Vitamin C, Ninja Red juice, Super-Cal, the following items are not manufactured by Young Living and made by Socar's Folic Acid and Carlson's Super Omega-3 Fish Oil. As mentioned in month 1, I continued to try and eat a healthier diet. Please speak to a licensed, trained professional for updated recommendations for supplements.

MONTH 6

I would awake in the middle of the night with numbness in my hands. A mild case of Carpal Syndrome turned venomous. I would lay with my hands by my sides and never above my head.

The sixth month of my pregnancy when I began to visualize the day of delivery. I wondered if the delivery would be painful? I jokingly tried to convince women to have my baby for me, but for some unknown reason they just wouldn't do it. I kept contemplating the possibility that I might need a C-section? Maybe I could just be a hermit, and the stork would deliver my baby?

THIRD TRIMESTER

MONTH 7

During the 7th month of my pregnancy, I saw Dr. Maxfield, and she performed an adjustment using acupuncture techniques as a means to prevent birth defects. Also, I continued taking folic acid to help prevent birth defects. I wanted to be certain that my baby was born healthy, and the acupuncture, changes in my diet and nutrition, including the folic acid and other supplements were all a part of the overall plan. I needed help to ensure the health of my baby.

> **A note from Dr. Maxfield regarding the use of acupuncture and chiropractic medicine during my pregnancy**
>
> Now, that you have heard about the success Andrea achieved from conception to birth of her "Miracle Baby" I am sure that you would like a quick lesson in how chiropractic and acupuncture work in balancing the human body. Let me start by explaining the stages of pathology, or disease. First, you have the cause, which then leads to disordered function. Only once the function is disrupted will you begin to see any symptoms. Once the symptoms appear, you will likely have disintegration or even organ failure depending on the disease. This means that many times you are already sick before you have any symptoms. As a matter of fact, I display a sign at my office letting people know that it is easier to stay well than to get well. During my acupuncture studies, I learned from traditional Chinese medicine that there are four aspects of health. The first aspect of health is acupuncture. They believe in healing not only on the physical level but also on the emotional and spiritual level. After acupuncture, they believe that to achieve optimal health, you must also have the spine in alignment, as well as have proper nutrition with herbal supplementation, as well as healthy mind-body balance. I know it Sounds very simple but, considering our lifestyle today, that may be easier said than done.

Simply put, acupuncture uses what is called meridians to balance out the energy levels within the body. No one can say for certain how acupuncture works, but we have seen even in the instances in this book that it can have a definite effect on the human body. What we do know is that acupuncture has a positive effect on the hypothalamus and pituitary gland releasing endorphins into the central nervous system to reduce pain. Many believe that endorphins are far more powerful than pain medications. It also believed that acupuncture changes the brain chemistry, as well as involuntary body functions. Basically, acupuncture can be used in a few different ways. The first is the simple use of pain control, in which the needles are placed over the area of pain. Secondly, an acupuncturist may use a formula somewhat like a recipe to treat a certain condition. Lastly, a traditional method may be used, which is formulated to balance out the meridians.

Chiropractic is somewhat similar because the manipulation addresses the central nervous system. The spinal nerves exit the spinal column in between each and every vertebra. If a vertebra is out of alignment the only way to restore function to that nerve is to re-align the bone. Different spinal nerves serve different functions. Some may help with arm or leg movement. The one thing that is important to understand is that some of the spinal nerves serve very important internal organs. If a nerve that supplies an internal organ is pinched, proper communication between the organ and the brain is not possible. Let me give you a couple of simple examples. Pretend that you have a water hose that is supplying water to your beautiful flower garden. Now, imagine that you accidentally step on the water hose. What will happen to your flowers? Yes, they will survive, but may suffer because they are not getting as much water as they need to flourish. Suppose now that you have a nasty, mean neighbor that does not like the beauty of your flowers and cuts the water hose in two. Of course now your flowers will die, right? Now, it is common for a spinal nerve to be completely severed. However, this is what can happen in some cases cause paralysis. Most common though is the analogy of just a kink in the hose. You still have a function, but not a function at 100 percent. This is the point when the body is open to possibly having some disease or illness. I believe that this is what happened in Andrea's case.

So, how do chiropractic and acupuncture work together? The simple answer and the one that I believe the most is that together they prevent disease in the first place. Together, they can also treat disease, the immune system, and stress. As someone who regularly receives both on a maintenance basis, I believe that they also improve the quality of life while promoting the longevity. Lastly, they can develop latent potentialities. I would encourage anyone who chooses to stay well to have a spinal checkup, as there may be things developing that have not manifested as symptoms.

I believe that most birth defects can be prevented by balancing the body and exercising prior to and during pregnancy, but you should always check with your doctor, practitioner, or nurse. I view my body as an incubator that must be fortified. I also believe a mother can do everything necessary to have a healthy child, but she and her partner must also consider the quality of the sperm as well as the health of the father.

TIP: In the early months of your pregnancy you should ask your doctor how much iron is necessary for pregnancy.

Note: Every day, I continually apply the hormone cream Progessence and take natural supplements from Young Living: Master Hers multivitamin, Vitamin C, Ninja Red juice, Super-Cal, and the following items not manufactured by Young Living and made by Socar's Folic Acid, Carlson's Super Omega-3 Fish Oil and *Socar's Iron*. As mentioned in month 1, I continued to try and eat a healthier diet. Please speak to a licensed, trained professional for updated recommendations for supplements.

During my 7th month, I had a difficult time sleeping. My sinuses were congested due to hay fever. The doctor said allergies were amplified during pregnancy. I'd wake up in the middle of the night unable to breath, but I'd remind myself that the discomfort was worth it.

This month we prepared our birthing plan. The book, *"What to Expect When You're Expecting"*, defines on page 274, "The typical plan combines the parents' wishes and preferences with that practitioner and hospital or birthing center find acceptable and what is feasible from a practical standpoint of view." Examples from the book, do you want an episiotomy, the use of forceps to deliver your baby or would you approve of a C-section?

We presented our birthing plan to my doctor. She said she would look it over and show it to her colleagues. The next month, she told me what we had planned was reasonable. I agreed. I saved a second copy for my husband, and I was saved for the big day, the night of November 6, 2006. And a third copy was given to the labor and delivery nurses accompanied by a box of chocolates or a basket of fruit.

MONTH 8

In the eighth month, I had my final monthly checkup with the doctor. Followed by four scheduled weekly visits in the ninth month visits or whatever my daughter decides to make her presence known. I continue to take all of my supplements.

> **Note: Every day, I continually apply the hormone cream Progessence and take natural supplements from Young Living: Master Hers multivitamin, Vitamin C, Ninja Red juice, Super-Cal, and the following items not manufactured by Young Living and made by Socar's Folic Acid, Carlson's Super Omega-3 Fish Oil and *Socar's Iron*. As mentioned in month 1, I continued to try and eat a healthier diet. Please speak to a licensed, trained professional for updated recommendations for supplements.**

Recently, we've heard the news that some vitamins aren't beneficial to our bodies. Magazines, the media have cited credible sources that Folic acid should be used to prevent birth defects. But, again, I'd also add acupuncture, chiropractic adjustments, cleansing the body, and Herbal wraps. I don't agree with not taking more vitamin C because my sister-in-law stated her fertility specialist prescribed more Vitamin C. Carl suggested the same thing to increase the Vitamin C to balance the body. Consider recent tests regarding Vitamin C, does the research specify what type or brand of a supplement was tested? The creation of this supplement was made from cayenne pepper, lemons, and grapefruits? Or was it, a supplement mainly mad from petroleum chemicals? Now, I use this rule: throw your supplement into a glass of water and see if it dissolves within 24 hours, 48 hours, or 72 hours? I ask myself, how healthy is a supplement that can't dissolve in water within 24 hours? Is it going into my bloodstream? Will I feel a benefit?

> **TIP:** The reason I went to Carl Janicek was to find out what supplements would balance or enhance all bodily functions. I envision a day when all doctors, trained medical personnel, homeopaths/naturopaths, chiropractors, acupuncturist, and dieticians will work together in a hospital facility, to prevent miscarriages, birth defects, and diseases.

The Young Living Vitamin C supplement I took daily through my pregnancy is called Super C. Notice the ingredients of Super C: Citrus Bioflavonoid, Rutin, Cayenne Pepper, Orange, Tangerine, Grapefruit, Lemon, and Lemongrass. Compare this to a regular grocery or drug store supplement. Remember, suggesting herbs to cleanse the intestines, and this was done to increase absorption of nutrients and supplements.

> **TIP:** After you have your child, check with your physician about reducing Vitamin C. Four months after my daughter's birth, I started experiencing heartburn. I spoke with a cardiologist, and she said to reduce the usage.

MONTH 9

This month I saw the Ob-gyn three times, it was to be four. Every visit this month they would check inside. I was swollen. It took two days to recover from the exam. Just prior to the exam they'd say, "Can you give us a urine sample? We need to check for protein in your urine." Okay. How can you possibly give them a decent sample, when you can't see past your feet, and you can't tell where to angle the cup—for the stream, because your child's head is resting on your bladder? I rolled along like a Rolly Polly bug! I started daydreaming that I must be in an episode from the past, "I Love Lucy", from the 50's. I must say, that I was embarrassed about the mere accident on the floor because I didn't tell anyone. Oops! Okay, please excuse my humor!

> **Note:** Every day, I continually apply the hormone cream Progessence and take natural supplements from Young Living: Master Hers multivitamin, Vitamin C, Ninja Red juice, Super-Cal, and the following items not manufactured by Young Living and made by Socar's Folic

Acid, Carlson's Super Omega-3 Fish Oil and *Socar's Iron*. As mentioned in month 1, I continued to try and eat a healthier diet. Please speak to a licensed, trained professional for updated recommendations for supplements.

I was so excited because I am just two weeks away from the due date. The doctor told me that if my daughter didn't make her presence known in two weeks that we could schedule an induction. I agreed. I was ready. The doctor scheduled the induction for November 6, 2006.

CONCLUSION

We arrived at the hospital on November 6, 2006, for the induction of my labor. The following day at 3:10 p.m., I was singing the lyrics to Helen Reddy' 1970 tune, "I am woman do you hear me roar", to myself, "It was I am woman, do you hear me scream? Oh my, lord, this is painful! Can I stop feeling like a bloated puffer fish?"

My husband, David (Dave) recalled vividly that the doctor had a hard time finding a heartbeat. She suggested a C-Section, as soon as possible. She informed him that there was a possibility the umbilical cord may be wrapped around our daughter's body.

Dave told me said that his first concern was that our baby might not make it. He was also concerned about my health. He remembers that the doctor donned him with a white medical cap and gown and a cap allowed him into the operating room, where he witnessed a bloody baby being lifted from my body. The doctor's assistant allowed my husband to cut the remaining cord; he recalled, and then, after a brief wash, the doctor's assistant handed him our brand new baby girl. My husband's exact words were, "I proudly showed Andrea, our new girl, and all Andrea could, say was, "Where was David, (thinking I was a staff member)?

I was groggy from the epidural, and I had cotton mouth. I looked to my left and thought it was the doctor. I heard this, "Honey". I realized this was my husband, and he was holding our beautiful baby girl with big brown eyes, and she was bald. She was a long and lanky child, 19 inches long and weighed 6 lbs. 3 oz. And, then my husband and I overheard the doctor say, "Happy Birthday, Baby!" I was unable to hold our beautiful baby girl because of the incision required for the C-Section.

"Aly" was delivered on at 3:15 p.m. on Election Day November 7, 2006. Shortly after all the celebration, the staff placed the pink cap on her head and wrapped her in the infamous burrito wrap with a baby blanket. I thought this day would never arrive. A day the likes of which I wish to all who read this story, and who will endure one of the most spectacular events of a lifetime.

So, maybe your journey started like mine, or maybe your situation is just a bit different than mine. I had had two miscarriages in my late 30's, so by this point, I realized I needed more help to sustain a healthy pregnancy. I needed to balance my entire body and to balance my hormones.

I saw my friend, Deanna Romero for a treatment during my second miscarriage. I needed Neuroenergetics to relax my body. This method of acupuncture is great because it works to eliminate the need for C-sections. Unfortunately, Deanna wasn't present at this pregnancy, and I did need a C-Section. But what made me consider the various methods of acupuncture is the fact it has existed for thousands and thousands of years in Asia. Can you imagine the research that could be done in Asia?

Also, regarding my second miscarriage, I saw the chiropractor/acupuncture/nurse two months before the second miscarriage. The chiropractor said in my third pregnancy, to come for my seventh-month adjustment and acupuncture to prevent birth defects.

Note: My daughter was standing up in my womb for the last two months of my pregnancy. After my daughter was a year old, she was delayed in walking, and she did need physical therapy until 23 months of age, and then she was off to the toddler races. At that time, the physical therapist believed her delay in walking was caused by my daughter standing up in the womb.

During my third and successful pregnancy, I saw Carl and Dr. Maxfield. Carl suggested cleansing my body again, but specifically the intestines. The intestines absorb nutrients, so it was imperative to get them functioning properly. While working with Carl, I learned I needed to take natural supplements, to eat healthier foods, to rest and to exercise for a successful pregnancy. In other words, I had to ramp up my body for my "Miracle Baby!"

I changed my diet for pregnancy, for the rest of my life, and for my child's life. I used to eat junk food about 50 percent of the time, or food of no nutritional value. So, I started eating more raw fruits, vegetables and freshly prepared foods a whopping 80 to 90 percent of the time. I also try to avoid foods cooked in a microwave, certain frozen foods loaded with chemicals I can't even pronounce. As well as foods made with bleached flour and white sugar, high fructose, hydrogenated fats, and corn syrup. I now have white chocolate lattes only four times a year. I did not drink alcoholic beverages during my pregnancy, although I drank non-alcoholic beverages. I now try to drink the standard amount of filtered water every day. I don't smoke. This was part of my preparation for a successful journey to motherhood. Again, I'm not perfect with my diet, so someone might occasionally see me eating a donut, but I only eat a donut once a month or not at all. I do believe in moderation.

> **TIP: Take both hormone creams prior to conception. Also, advise your doctor about what you're doing. Remember, the nurse told me to discontinue the Prenelone cream during pregnancy. She said I could continue using the hormone cream Progessence, which is a more natural hormonal supplement for progesterone. Please note the hormone creams aren't totally natural. Please talk to a licensed/trained professional for updated product recommendations.**
>
> **My suggestions for finding credible professionals for the following: herbal wraps, homeopaths/naturopaths, chiropractors and acupuncturists, include the following: contact your family doctor, find an ob-gyn, contact spas, managers of health food stores, and massage therapists. In your state check their records with the Better Business Bureau. If you live in a remote area, consider traveling to the nearest major city. Also, you can use Google, Metacrawler, Yahoo, Twitter, Ask, and Facebook.**

Finally, I am excited for all of you who want to conceive a healthy child, but first we must consider our environment, our legal system, and that acupuncture works.

It worked for me, but to make it work more effectively or efficiently, I balanced my body, and I exercised consistently and regularly (or often). I believe laws in this country should protect women in the workplace during pregnancy and advocate for changes to be made. They should also protect both the woman and her spouse/partner during pregnancy, menopause, and in the case of postpartum depression. Also, I dream of the day, when I will walk into any hospital and see/smell aroma- therapy being used by doctors and all medical personnel. Then exercise physiologists and cleanses should be used for healing processes. I also dream that one day soon we will all realize our balanced diet, our use of proper, healthy food is key to successful pregnancies, and to ending many diseases and illnesses in our society. Healthier food is produced by a healthy ecosystem because without it, in the future there will be no jobs and no children. Consider what my ancient, indigenous ancestors believed, "What we take from Mother Earth, and then we must put it back in its simplest form. Heal Mother Earth, heal yourself!" An unhealthy environment creates a bad economy! I wish you and your children wealth, health, and happiness! So, I dedicate this song to all of you out there, "Ain't No Mountain High Enough," as sung by Diana Ross!

APPENDIX

Flow and Pathways of Disease:

Homeopathic perspectives and perceptions…

Health is an *Ease of Flow…* of

Blood, Breath, Water, Waste, Communications, Nerves, Love, Response Emotions, Nutrients, Energy, Abundance, etc.

I. **Primary causes** of disease… are violations of Natural Law and Blockages of flow resulting from:

Internal

1. Stress – Body, Mind, Spirit, Social and Environmental

2. Lack of Education and Awareness – Ignorance of …Body, Structural Imbalances, and Social or Environmental Messages

3. Mental Factors – Excess Anger, Grief, Anxiety, Greed, or, Lack or Suppression of Expression, etc.

4. Heredity – Bad or damaged genes and genetic expression resulting in increased decreased nutrient needs and environmental sensitivities

5. Allergic Reactivity – unregulated immune responses, improper dietary exposures, natural "blood type" or "Body Type" antigens and triggers

External

1. Toxicity – Synthetic and Auto-toxicity

2. Trauma – Micro or Major, physical or emotional

3. Pathogen – Micro-organism out its natural environment

4. Perverse Energy – Excess heat, cold, wind, humidity, noise, microwaves, electromagnetic radiation, ionizing radiation, x-ray, negative attitudes, etc.

5. Deficiency or excess nutrients – fatty acids, amino acids, vitamins, minerals, carbohydrates, preservatives, air, exercise, daylight, love, communications, friendship, intellectual stimulation, sense or personal value, productivity, etc.

II. Adaptation Syndrome – mostly symptom free

Functional Disturbance of Organs – imbalanced energetically and at cellular level

III. Exhaustion Phase – Organic Dysfunction in Physical Makeup of Organs (Inflamed or Degenerative)

IV. Death (Of Cells, Tissues, Organs, Organ systems or of the total organism)

V. Other natural causes of disease…

Nature of Miasms:

Psora – Fear based…Improper use of mental facilities, original disconnection from spiritual source, addicted to rationalizations and information to overcome fear…gives away energy to compensate, expression of poverty, consciousness physical and/or energetic…potential skin health issues. Psora is the grandfather of all diseases.

1. Psychosis-Control based…improper use of will, disregulation of systems, especially endocrine and mucosal systems, desire to control others energy or be controlled by others, while unable to controls themselves.

2. Syphilis – Action based…Improper use of actions founded on the desires and need to draw energy from outside of self…surroundings, including people, animals and natural systems. Syphilis-action based is attractive, seductive yet most destructive…and willing to die or to kill to protect their beliefs, self-image and material possessions.

INDEX

acupuncture and chiropractor, 14,17,24
acupuncture to prevent birth defects, 15
adequate weight loss, 17

birthing plan, 3
blood drawn, 8, 17
box of chocolates, 3

Carl Janicek, 23,24.25, 43
Carpal Tunnel, 60
Children of Men, 56
chiropractor and acupuncture, 14
conception, 7
C-Section, 3
Conclusion, 68

d and c, 7, 22
Deanna Romero, 4, 10
dehydrated, 12
Diana Ross sung, *"Ain't No Mountain High Enough,"*
High Enough, 8,
dilation, 3, 20
Dr. Adano, 29
Dr. Chavarro, 18
Dr. Maxfield, 14

epidural, 3, 6, 8

Fertility Diet, 18

Google Birthing Plan, 3

Herbal laxatives, 59
Herbal Wrap, 12, 13, 70
Herrings Law of Cure, 31

Inflammatory Pathology, 27
Intestines, 4

Janicek, Carl, 23, 66

K.C. and Sunshine Band, "Get Down Tonight", 13
Kegel Exercises, 18, 20

Law-Know it, 8
Liver Cleanse, 9

Men's Health, 43
Mermaid Wrap, 13
Meridians, 21, 25, 26
Misalignment of Pelvis, 19
Miscarriages 8, 9
Molar pregnancy 6, 16, 22
month 1, 54
month 2, 57
month 3, 58
month 4, 59
month 5, 59
month 6, 60
month 7, 62
month 8, 65
month 9, 66
mosquitoes, 60

nauseated, 12, 17
N.E.R., 19, 20
neuroenergetic, 19, 20

ovulation, 54
oxytocin, 3

pitocin, 3
ph balance 32
positive affirmation, 17
Prenelone, 55, 57, 58, 59, 60, 64
Progessence, 55, 57, 58, 59, 60
prune juice, 59

Deanna Romero, P.A., 18, 19, 20
sciatic nerve, 15
sperm count, 2
Stress, 18
Supplements, 55, 56, 57, 59, 60

"Taking Charge of Your Fertility, the Definitive Guide to Natural Birth Control,
Pregnancy Achievement, and Reproductive
Health, 6,7
Trimester 17, 54
Trimester 2, 59
Trimester 3, 62
Tsing points, 26

ultrasound, 7, 21, 22
urine sample, 18

Victoria Secret, 22
Vitamins, 65

"What to expect when you're expecting," by Heidi Murkoff, Arlene Eisenburg, and Sandee Hathaway B.S.N., 57, 64

Young Living (youngliving.com), 26, 56

BIBLIOGRAPHY

Adamo, Dr., Peter J. *Eat Right 4 Your Type*. New York: G.P. Putnam's Sons, 1996. (Carl's)

Chavarro MD, ScD, Jorge E. and Willett MD, DrPH, Walter. *The Fertility Diet*. New York:
McGraw Hill Publishing Co., 2007.

Desk Reference. *Essential Oils*. 2nd Edition. United States of America. (Carl's)
Herring

K.C. and the Sunshine Band. *Get Down Tonight*.

Mein D.C., Carolyn L. *Releasing Emotional Patterns with Essential Oils*. Fifth Edition. Rancho Santa Fe, Ca.: Vision Ware Press, 2004. (Carl's)

Murkoff, Heidi, Arlene Eisenberg, Sandee Hathaway, B.S.N. *What to Expect When You're*
Expecting. New York: Workman Publishing Co., 2002.

Reddy, Helen. *I am Woman, Do you hear me roar?*

Ross, Diana. *Ain't No Mountain High Enough*.

The movie, *Children of Men*.

Weschler, Toni. *Taking Charge of Your Fertility: the Definitive Guide to Natural Birth Control,*
Pregnancy Achievement, and Reproductive Health. New York: Harper Collins Publishers,
Inc., 2002.

Wiley Phd, Rudolf A. *Biobalance, the Acid/Alkaline Solution to the Food-Mood-Health Puzzle*.
Utah: Essential Science Publishing, 1989. (Carl's)

Yasgur, R. Ph., M.Sc. Jay. *A Dictionary of Homeopathic Medical Terminology.* 3rd Edition.
Greenville, Pa.: Van Hoy Publishers. (Carl's Hering and homepath terms, Organon)

Young N.D., D. Gary. *Re-JUVA-nate Your Health: Liver Cleanse.* 2003 Young Living Oils.

ABOUT THE AUTHORS

Andrea Duran-Carpenter: She holds a B.A. in Communications, a minor in Health Fitness Education, and an MBA with an emphasis in Marketing. She is pursuing second Master's Degree in Special Education. She currently, resides in Colorado. She was inspired to write this book to acknowledge the women who contributed to her story and of the successful birth of her daughter, and because of the professionals and authors who aided in this journey.

Carl Janicek: He worked at Craig Hospital in Englewood, Colorado. There he learned a great deal about the current medical model being used in rehabilitation work, patient care, occupational therapy, speech therapy, and emergency procedures.

Dr. Janicek studied acupuncture in more depth under Dr. Eric Tao, O.M.D., including 1200 hours of classes. He decided acupuncture was not the first choice of how he'd like to spend his time. In the 80's, he was enthralled to utilize the Chinese philosophies and pursued a Bachelor of Science degree in Wellness Nutrition, a pastoral degree. He was then persuaded by Dr. William Nelson N.D., to consider a scientific view of Homeopathy, and he finished his Doctorate of Homeopathy.

Dr. Stacey Maxfield, D.C., and B.S.N.: She was born and raised in Iowa. The summer before her senior year in high school, her father took a severance package from John Deere. Their family then moved to Texas. She has her doctorate from the Parker College of Chiropractic, located in Dallas Texas. Due to the extreme heat in that state and the lack of outdoor activities, she moved to Colorado. There she continued her education with the study of acupuncture. Eventually, she added that practice to her license. This wonderful, compassionate, and talented doctor, passed on August 9, 2012, to breast cancer. She was just shy of her forty-first birthday. She is missed. God bless her, and may the world know and understand her passion, the benefits to all humanity: Chiropractic and Acupuncture! Thank you, for everything! Thank you, to her husband, Eric Meister, and daughter Zoe Meister! Please note, a portion of proceeds from this book, will be donated to the Susan G. Komen Foundation in memory of Dr. Stacey Maxfield.

Deanna Romero, P.A.: She started her medical journey as a child. In her family, she was the one who cared for their wounded and sick animals. She started learning massage therapy at a young age. Her father had a herniated disk, so he always selected Deanna to massage his back. He would mention how strong her hands were. She always had this desire to help people; therefore, she pursued a career in the health profession. Soon she discovered the limitations of Western Medicine.

Romero became a Physician Assistant (PA) in 1990 upon graduation from the University of Colorado Health Science Center (UCHSC), in the Child Health Associate Program. She also obtained a Master's degree from UCHSC. She has a wealth of knowledge in medicine, with Pediatrics being her primary specialty along with Adolescent Medicine, Obstetrics and Gynecology, Trauma, and Adult Primary Care.

It was during her first year in the Physician Assistant (P.A.) School when she was introduced to Alternative Medicine. She was writing a paper on "Curanerismo," which is about Mexican traditional folk healers. She was interviewing a "Curandera," a friend of the family, who then presented Romero with an offer to study with her. Romero was honored but had to decline due to the rigorous P.A. Programs. She had at the time her son was a Dentist, who had diagnosed her with TMJ, a fact she shared with this "Curandera." She recommended Romero should see her niece who performed Neuromuscular Massage. So she went to see this woman who helped her in more ways than just a neuromuscular massage. The niece was a very gifted lady who not only helped people physically, but emotionally, and spiritually. Romero now refers to her as a modernized "Curandera," who exposed her to Young Living Essential Oils, which she used in combination with her body work. Romero was fascinated with these oils and has been studying Aroma Therapy ever since.

During the last ten years, Romero has become more disciplined with the use of these oils. She shares them with her family and friends, when they call her about different health conditions, sometimes asking for a prescription, which is unethical. Therefore, she offers some combination of essential oils that takes care of the problem. On her journey to learn about essential oils, she met another healer who took her to another level with oils and introduced her to Neuro-energetic Release Therapy (NER). This healer convinced her to take this course. The instructor was a little skeptical about allowing her to take his course. But once she explained to him her findings from her work as a P.A. on people with back pain, and associating other problems related to back pain, such as TMJ, Plantar Fasciitis, headaches and so forth, he decided to let her take the course.

She has been applying the techniques of NER for almost eight years now, which has been one of the most gratifying aspects of her ability to help people. To know she does not have to give them prescriptions and then say, "Take these meds, and if you are not better in two weeks or get worse, come back to see me," is important to her. She has been successful helping people with a variety of problems, such as all types of back pain (including growing pains). She has also performed a large amount of injury prevention work. This work was done without the use medications. As for her personal healing, her work has eliminated her previously frequent trips to the Chiropractor and Message Therapist. Two NER treatment's a year now keep her body balanced and pain-free.

www.ingramcontent.com/pod-product-compliance
Lightning Source LLC
Chambersburg PA
CBHW081829170526
45167CB00007B/2760